Virtual Clinical Excursions—Obstetrics

for

Lowdermilk and Perry:
Maternity and Women's Health Care,
8th Edition

Virtual Clinical Excursions—Obstetrics

for

Lowdermilk and Perry:
Maternity and Women's Health Care,
8th Edition

prepared by

Kitty Cashion, RN, BC, MSN
Clinical Nurse Specialist
University of Tennessee, Memphis, Health Science Center
Department of Obstetrics and Gynecology
Division of Maternal-Fetal Medicine
Memphis, Tennessee

Kelly Ann Crum, RN, MSN
Instructional Specialist
Lead Faculty
Curriculum Development/Maternal Child Nursing Specialty
Health Sciences and Nursing Department
University of Phoenix, Online
Phoenix, Arizona

software developed by

Wolfsong Informatics, LLC
Tucson, Arizona

ELSEVIER
MOSBY

ELSEVIER
MOSBY

11830 Westline Industrial Dr.
St. Louis, Missouri 63146

VIRTUAL CLINICAL EXCURSIONS—OBSTETRICS FOR   ISBN 0-323-03037-8
LOWDERMILK AND PERRY: MATERNITY AND WOMEN'S HEALTH CARE
EIGHTH EDITION
Copyright © 2006, Mosby, Inc.

Although for mechanical reasons all pages of this publication are perforated, only those pages imprinted with a Mosby, Inc. copyright notice are intended for removal.

Notice

Knowledge and best practice in this field are constantly changing. As new research and experience broaden our knowledge, changes in practice, treatment and drug therapy may become necessary or appropriate. Readers are advised to check the most current information provided (i) on procedures featured or (ii) by the manufacturer of each product to be administered, to verify the recommended dose or formula, the method and duration of administration, and contraindications. It is the responsibility of the practitioner, relying on their own experience and knowledge of the patient, to make diagnoses, to determine dosages and the best treatment for each individual patient, and to take all appropriate safety precautions. To the fullest extent of the law, neither the Publisher nor the Authors assumes any liability for any injury and/or damage to persons or property arising out or related to any use of the material contained in this book.

International Standard Book Number 0-323-03037-8

Senior Editor, Nursing: *Tom Wilhelm*
Managing Editor: *Jeff Downing*
Associate Developmental Editor: *Jennifer Anderson*
Project Manager: *Joy Moore*

Printed in the United States of America

Last digit is the print number: 9 8 7 6 5 4 3 2 1

*Workbook
prepared by*

Kitty Cashion, RN, BC, MSN
Clinical Nurse Specialist
University of Tennessee, Memphis, Health Science Center
Department of Obstetrics and Gynecology
Division of Maternal-Fetal Medicine
Memphis, Tennessee

Kelly Ann Crum, RN, MSN
Instructional Specialist
Lead Faculty
Curriculum Development/Maternal Child Nursing Specialty
Health Sciences and Nursing Department
University of Phoenix, Online
Phoenix, Arizona

Textbook

Deitra Leonard Lowdermilk, RNC, PhD, FAAN
Clinical Professor, School of Nursing
University of North Carolina at Chapel Hill
Chapel Hill, North Carolina

Shannon E. Perry, RN, CNS, PhD, FAAN
Professor, School of Nursing
San Francisco State University
San Francisco, California

Contents

Getting Started

Getting Set Up 1
A Quick Tour 9
A Detailed Tour 24

Unit I—Introduction to Maternity and Women's Health Nursing

Lesson 1   Community Care: The Family and Culture (Chapter 2) 43
Lesson 2   Assessment and Health Promotion (Chapter 5) 51

Unit II—Women's Health

Lesson 3   Violence Against Women (Chapter 6) 57
Lesson 4   Reproductive System Concerns, Contraception, and Infertility
            (Chapters 7, 9, and 10) 65
Lesson 5   Sexually Transmitted and Other Infections (Chapter 8) 71

Unit III—Pregnancy

Lesson 6   Assessment of Risk Factors in Pregnancy,
            Including Maternal and Fetal Nutrition (Chapters 15 and 29) 77
Lesson 7   Nursing Care During Pregnancy (Chapter 16) 83

Unit IV—Childbirth

Lesson 8   Nursing Care During Labor and Birth (Chapter 21) 89
Lesson 9   Management of Discomfort (Chapter 19) 97

Unit V—Complications of Pregnancy

Lesson 10   Hypertensive Disorders in Pregnancy (Chapter 30) 107
Lesson 11   Antepartal Hemorrhagic Disorders (Chapter 32) 113
Lesson 12   Endocrine and Metabolic Disorders (Chapter 32) 121
Lesson 13   Medical-Surgical Problems in Pregnancy (Chapter 33) 129
Lesson 14   Mental Health Disorders and Substance Abuse (Chapter 35) 137
Lesson 15   Labor and Birth Complications (Chapter 36) 145

Unit VI—Newborn Complications

Lesson 16   Newborn Complications (Chapters 38 and 40) 153
Lesson 17   Grieving the Loss of a Newborn (Chapter 41) 163

Unit VII—Medications in Obstetrics

Lesson 18   Medication Administration 167

Contents

Table of Contents
Lowdermilk and Perry:
Maternity and Women's Health Care, 8th Edition

Unit 1 Introduction to Maternity and Women's Health Care

1 Contemporary Maternity Nursing and Women's Health Care
2 Community Care: The Family and Culture (Lesson 1)
3 Genetics
4 Alternative and Complementary Therapies

Unit 2 Women's Health

5 Assessment and Health Promotion (Lesson 2)
6 Violence Against Women (Lesson 3)
7 Reproductive System Concerns (Lesson 4)
8 Sexually Transmitted and Other Infections (Lesson 5)
9 Contraception and Abortion (Lesson 4)
10 Infertility (Lesson 4)
11 Problems of the Breast
12 Structural Disorders and Neoplasms of the Reproductive System

Unit 3 Pregnancy

13 Conception and Fetal Development
14 Anatomy and Physiology of Pregnancy
15 Maternal and Fetal Nutrition (Lesson 6)
16 Nursing Care During Pregnancy (Lesson 7)
17 Childbirth and Perinatal Education

Unit 4 Childbirth

18 Labor and Birth Processes
19 Management of Discomfort (Lesson 9)
20 Fetal Assessment During Labor
21 Nursing Care During Labor (Lesson 8)

Unit 5 Postpartum

22 Postpartum Physiology
23 Nursing Care of the Postpartum Woman
24 Transition to Parenthood

Unit 6 The Newborn

25 Physiologic and Behavioral Adaptations of the Newborn
26 Nursing Care of the Newborn
27 Newborn Nutrition and Feeding
28 Care of the Newborn at Home

Unit 7   Complications of Pregnancy

29   Assessment for Risk Factors (Lesson 6)
30   Hypertensive Disorders in Pregnancy (Lesson 10)
31   Antepartal Hemorrhagic Disorders
32   Endocrine and Metabolic Disorders (Lesson 11 and 12)
33   Medical-Surgical Problems in Pregnancy (Lesson 13)
34   Obstetric Critical Care
35   Mental Health Disorders and Substance Abuse (Lesson 14)
36   Labor and Birth Complications (Lesson 15)
37   Postpartum Complications

Unit 8   Newborn Complications

38   Acquired Problems of the Newborn (Lesson 16)
39   Hemolytic Disorders and Congenital Anomalies
40   Nursing Care of the High-Risk Newborn (Lesson 16)
41   Grieving the Loss of a Newborn (Lesson 17)

Getting Started

GETTING SET UP

■ MINIMUM SYSTEM REQUIREMENTS

WINDOWS™

Windows XP, 2000, 98, ME, NT 4.0 (Recommend Windows XP/2000)
Pentium® III processor (or equivalent) @ 600 MHz (Recommend 800 MHz or better)
128 MB of RAM (Recommend 256 MB or more)
800 x 600 screen size (Recommend 1024 x 768)
Thousands of colors
12x CD-ROM drive
Soundblaster 16 soundcard compatibility
Stereo speakers or headphones

Note: Virtual Clinical Excursions—Obstetrics for Windows will require a minimal amount of disk space to install icons and required dll files for Windows 98/ME.

MACINTOSH®

MAC OS X (10.2 or higher)
Apple Power PC G3 @ 500 MHz or better
128 MB of RAM (Recommend 256 MB or more)
800 x 600 screen size (Recommend 1024 x 768)
Thousands of colors
12x CD-ROM drive
Stereo speakers or headphones

■ INSTALLATION INSTRUCTIONS

WINDOWS

1. Insert the *Virtual Clinical Excursions—Obstetrics* CD-ROM.
2. Inserting the CD should automatically bring up the setup screen if the current product is not already installed.
   a. If the setup screen does not appear automatically (and *Virtual Clinical Excursions—Obstetrics* has not been installed already), navigate to the "My Computer" icon on your desktop or in your Start menu.
   b. Double-click on your CD-ROM drive.
   c. If installation does not start at this point:
      (1) Click the **Start** icon on the task bar and select the **Run** option.
      (2) Type d:\setup.exe (where "d:\" is your CD-ROM drive) and press **OK**.
      (3) Follow the onscreen instructions for installation.
3. Follow the onscreen instructions during the setup process.

MACINTOSH

1. Insert the *Virtual Clinical Excursions—Obstetrics* CD in the CD-ROM drive. The disk icon will appear on your desktop.

2. Double-click on the disk icon.

3. Double-click on the OBSTETRICS_MAC run file.

NOTE: *Virtual Clinical Excursions—Obstetrics* for Macintosh does not have an installation setup and can only be run directly from the CD.

■ HOW TO USE VIRTUAL CLINICAL EXCURSIONS—OBSTETRICS

WINDOWS

1. Double-click on the *Virtual Clinical Excursions—Obstetrics* icon located on your desktop.
2. Or navigate to the program via the Windows Start menu.

NOTE: Windows 98/ME will require you to restart your computer before running the *Virtual Clinical Excursions—Obstetrics* program.

MACINTOSH

1. Insert the *Virtual Clinical Excursions—Obstetrics* CD in the CD-ROM drive. The disk icon will appear on your desktop.

2. Double-click on the disk icon.

3. Double-click on the OBSTETRICS_MAC run file.

■ SCREEN SETTINGS

For best results, your computer monitor resolution should be set at a minimum of 800 x 600. The number of colors displayed should be set to "thousands or higher" (High Color or 16 bit) or "millions of colors" (True Color or 24 bit).

Windows™

1. From the **Start** menu, select **Control Panel** (on some systems, you will first go to **Settings**, then to **Control Panel**).
2. Double-click on the **Display** icon.
3. Click on the **Settings** tab.
4. Under **Screen area** use the slider bar to select **800 by 600 pixels**.
5. Access the **Colors** drop-down menu by clicking on the down arrow.
6. Select **High Color (16 bit)** or **True Color (24 bit)**.
7. Click on **OK**.
8. You may be asked to verify the setting changes. Click **Yes**.
9. You may be asked to restart your computer to accept the changes. Click **Yes**.

Macintosh®

1. Select the **Monitors** control panel.
2. Select **800 x 600** (or similar) from the **Resolution** area.
3. Select **Thousands** or **Millions** from the **Color Depth** area.

■ WEB BROWSERS

Supported web browsers include Microsoft Internet Explorer (IE) version 5.0 or higher and Netscape version 4.5 or higher. *Note that Netscape version 6.0 is not supported at this time, although versions 6.2 and higher are supported.*

If you use America Online (AOL) for web access, you will need AOL version 4.0 or higher and IE 5.0 or higher. Do not use earlier versions of AOL with earlier versions of IE, because you will have difficulty accessing many features.

For best results with AOL:
- Connect to the Internet using AOL version 4.0 or higher.
- Open a private chat within AOL (this allows the AOL client to remain open, without asking whether you wish to disconnect while minimized).
- Minimize AOL.
- Launch a recommended browser.

■ TECHNICAL SUPPORT

Technical support for this product is available between 7:30 a.m. and 7 p.m. CST, Monday through Friday. Before calling, be sure that your computer meets the minimum system requirements to run this software. Inside the United States and Canada, call 1-800-692-9010. Outside North America, call 314-872-8370. You may also fax your questions to 314-997-5080 or contact Technical Support through e-mail: technical.support@elsevier.com.

Trademarks: Windows, Macintosh, Pentium, and America Online are registered trademarks.

ACCESSING *Virtual Clinical Excursions—Obstetrics* FROM EVOLVE

The product you have purchased is part of the Evolve family of online courses and learning resources. Please read the following information completely to get started.

To access your instructor's course on Evolve:

Your instructor will provide you with the username and password needed to access their specific course on the Evolve Learning System. Once you have received this information, please follow these instructions:

1. Go to the Evolve student page (http://evolve.elsevier.com/student)

2. Enter your username and password in the **Login to My Evolve** area and click the **Login** button.

3. You will be taken to your personalized **My Evolve** page where the course will be listed in the **My Courses** module.

TECHNICAL REQUIREMENTS

To use an Evolve course, you will need access to a computer that is connected to the Internet and equipped with web browser software that supports frames. For optimal performance, it is recommended that you have speakers and use a high-speed Internet connection. However, slower dial-up modems (56 K minimum) are acceptable.

Whichever browser you use, the browser preferences must be set to enable cookies and Java/JavaScript and the cache must be set to reload every time.

Enable Cookies

Browser	Steps
Internet Explorer 5.0 or higher	1. Select **Tools**. 2. Select **Internet Options**. 3. Select **Security** tab. 4. Make sure **Internet** (globe) is highlighted. 5. Select **Custom Level** button. 6. Scroll down the **Security Settings** list. 7. Under **Cookies** heading, make sure **Enable** is selected. 8. Click **OK**.
Internet Explorer 6.0	1. Select **Tools**. 2. Select **Internet Options**. 3. Select **Privacy** tab. 4. Use the slider (slide down) to **Accept All Cookies**. 5. Click **OK**. -OR- 4. Click the **Advanced** button. 5. Click the check box next to **Override Automatic Cookie Handling**. 6. Click the **Accept** buttons under **First-party Cookies** and **Third-party Cookies**. 7. Click **OK**.
Netscape Communicator or Navigator 4.5 or higher	1. Select **Edit**. 2. Select **Preferences**. 3. Click **Advanced**. 4. Click **Accept all cookies**. 5. Click **OK**.
Netscape Communicator or Navigator 6.1 or higher	1. Select **Edit**. 2. Select **Preferences**. 3. Select **Privacy & Security**. 4. Select **Cookies**. 5. Select **Enable All Cookies**.

Enable Java

Browser	Steps
Internet Explorer 5.0 or higher	1. Select **Tools**. 2. Select **Internet Options**. 3. Select the **Advanced** tab. 4. Locate **Microsoft VM**. 5. Make sure the **Java console enabled** and **Java logging enabled** boxes are checked. 6. Click **OK**. 7. Restart your computer if you checked the **Java console enabled** box.
Netscape Communicator or Navigator 4.5 or higher	1. Select **Edit** 2. Select **Preferences**. 3. Select **Advanced**. 4. Make sure the **Enable Java** and **Enable JavaScript** boxes are checked. 5. Click **OK**.

Set Cache to Always Reload a Page

Browser	Steps
Internet Explorer 5.0 or higher	1. Select **Tools**. 2. Select **Internet Options**. 3. Select the **General** tab. 4. Select **Settings** from within the **Temporary Internet Files** section. 5. Select the **Every visit to the page** button. 6. Click **OK**.
Netscape Communicator or Navigator 4.5 or higher	1. Select **Edit** 2. Select **Preferences**. 2. Click the + or → icon next to the **Advanced** to see more options. 3. Select **Cache**. 4. Select the **Every time** button at the bottom. 5. Click **OK**.

Plug-Ins

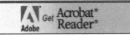 **Adobe Acrobat Reader**—With the free Acrobat Reader software you can view and print Adobe PDF files. Many Evolve products offer student and instructor manuals, checklists, and more in this format!

Download at: http://www.adobe.com

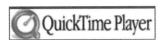 **Apple QuickTime**—Install this to hear word pronunciations, heart and lung sounds, and many other helpful audio clips within Evolve Online Courses!

Download at: http://www.apple.com

 Macromedia Flash Player—This player will enhance your viewing of many Evolve web pages, as well as educational short-form to long-form animation within the Evolve Learning System!

Download at: http://www.macromedia.com

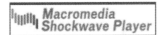 **Macromedia Shockwave Player**—Shockwave is best for viewing the many interactive learning activities within Evolve Online Courses!

Download at: http: //www.macromedia.com

 Microsoft Word Viewer—With this viewer Microsoft Word users can share documents with those who don't have Word, and users without Word can open and view Word documents. Many Evolve products have testbank, student and instructor manuals, and other documents available for downloading and viewing on your own computer!

Download at: http://www.microsoft.com

 Microsoft PowerPoint Viewer—View PowerPoint 97, 2000, and 2002 presentations even if you don't have PowerPoint with this viewer. Many Evolve products have slides available for downloading and viewing on your own computer!

Download at: http://www.microsoft.com

SUPPORT INFORMATION

Live support is available to customers in the United States and Canada from 7:30 a.m. to 7:00 p.m. (Central Time), Monday through Friday by calling, **1-800-401-9962**. You can also send an email to evolve-support@elsevier.com.

There is also **24/7 support information** available on the Evolve website (http://evolve.elsevier.com), including:

- Guided Tours
- Tutorials
- Frequently Asked Questions (FAQs)
- Online Copies of Course User Guides
- And much more!

A QUICK TOUR

Welcome to *Virtual Clinical Excursions—Obstetrics*, a virtual hospital setting in which you can work with multiple complex patient simulations and also learn to access and evaluate the information resources that are essential for high-quality patient care.

The virtual hospital, Pacific View Regional Hospital, has realistic architecture and access to patient rooms, a Nurses' Station, and a Medication Room.

■ BEFORE YOU START

Make sure you have your textbook nearby when you use the *Virtual Clinical Excursions—Obstetrics* CD. You will want to consult topic areas in your textbook frequently while working with the CD and using this workbook.

■ HOW TO SIGN IN

- First, enter your name on the Student Nurse identification badge.
- Now select a period of care. The screen gives you four periods of care from which to choose. In Periods of Care 1 through 3, you can actively engage in patient assessment, entry of data in the electronic patient record (EPR), and medication administration. Period of Care 4 presents the day in review. Click on the appropriate period of care. (For this quick tour, choose **Period of Care 2**.)
- This takes you to the Patient List screen (see example on page 11). Note that the virtual time is provided in the box at the lower left corner of the screen (1115, since we chose Period of Care 2).

Note: If you choose to work during Period of Care 4: 1900-2000, the Patient List screen will not appear since you are not able to visit patients or administer medications during the shift. Instead, you are taken directly to the Nurses' Station, where the records of all the patients on the floor are available for your review.

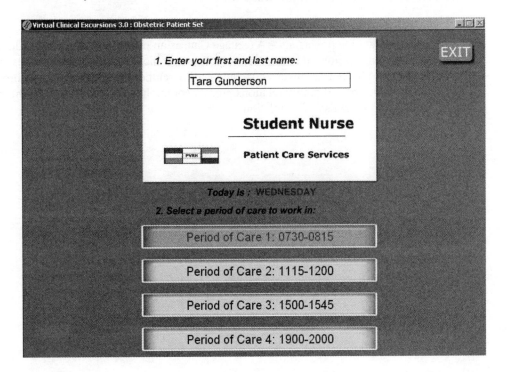

■ **PATIENT LIST**

OBSTETRICS UNIT

Dorothy Grant (Room 201)
30-week intrauterine pregnancy—A young Caucasian multipara admitted with abdominal trauma following a domestic violence incident. Her complications include preterm labor and extensive social issues such as acquiring safe housing for her family upon discharge.

Stacey Crider (Room 202)
27-week intrauterine pregnancy—A young Native American primigravida admitted for intravenous tocolysis, bacterial vaginosis, and poorly controlled insulin-dependent gestational diabetes. Strained family relationships and social isolation complicate this patient's ability to comply with strict dietary requirements and prenatal care.

Kelly Brady (Room 203)
26-week intrauterine pregnancy—A 35-year-old Caucasian primigravida urgently admitted for progressive symptoms of preeclampsia. A history of inadequate coping with major life stressors leave her at risk for a recurrence of depression as she faces a diagnosis of HELLP syndrome and the delivery of a severely premature infant.

Maggie Gardner (Room 204)
22-week intrauterine pregnancy—A 41-year-old African-American multigravida admitted for a high-risk pregnancy evaluation and rule out diagnosis of systemic lupus erythematosus. Coping with chronic pain, fatigue, and a history of multiple miscarriages contribute to an anxiety disorder and the need for social service intervention.

Gabriela Valenzuela (Room 205)
34-week intrauterine pregnancy—A young Hispanic primigravida with a history of mitral valve prolapse admitted for uterine cramping and vaginal bleeding suggestive of placental abruption following an unrestrained motor vehicle accident. Her needs include staff support for an unprepared-for labor and possible preterm birth.

Laura Wilson (Room 206)
37-week intrauterine pregnancy—A teenage Caucasian primigravida urgently admitted after being found unconscious at home. Her complications include HIV-positive status and chronic polysubstance abuse. Unrealistic expectations of parenthood and living with a chronic illness combined with strained family relations prompt comprehensive social and psychiatric evaluations initiated on the day of simulation.

■ HOW TO SELECT A PATIENT

- You can choose one or more patients to work with from the Patient List by clicking the box to the left of the patient name(s). (In order to receive a scorecard for a patient, the patient must be selected before proceeding to the Nurses' Station.)
- Click on **Get Report** to the right of the medical records number (MRN) to view a summary of the patient's care during the 12-hour period before your arrival on the unit.
- After reviewing the report, click on **Return to Patient List**.
- When you are ready to begin your care, click on **Go to Nurses' Station** in the right lower corner.

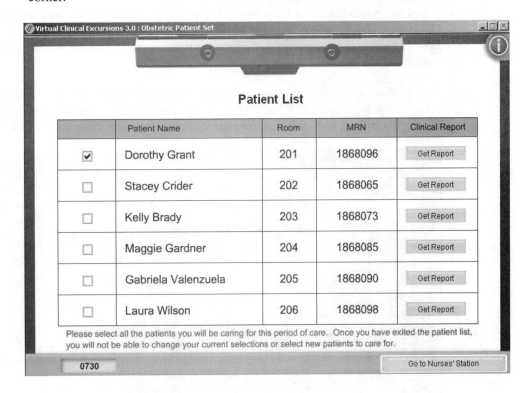

■ HOW TO FIND A PATIENT'S RECORDS

NURSES' STATION

Within the Nurses' Station, you will see:

1. A clipboard that contains the patient list for that floor.
2. A chart rack with patient charts labeled by room number, a notebook labeled Kardex, and a notebook labeled MAR (Medication Administration Record).
3. A desktop computer with access to the Electronic Patient Record (EPR).
4. A tool bar across the top of the screen that can also be used to access the Patient List, EPR, Chart, MAR, and Kardex. This tool bar is also accessible from each patient's room.
5. A Drug Guide containing information about the medications you are able to administer to your patients.

As you run your cursor over an item, it will be highlighted. To select, simply double-click on the item. As you use these resources, you will always be able to return to the Nurses' Station by clicking on the **Return to Nurses' Station** bar located in the right lower corner of your screen.

MEDICATION ADMINISTRATION RECORD (MAR)

The MAR icon located in the tool bar at the top of your screen accesses current 24-hour medications for each patient. Click on the icon and the MAR will open. (*Note:* You can also access the MAR by clicking on the blue MAR notebook on the far right side of the book rack in the center of the screen.) Within the MAR, tabs on the right side of the screen allow you to select patients by room number. Be careful to make sure you select the correct tab number for *your* patient rather than simply reading the first record that appears after the MAR opens. Each MAR sheet lists the following:

- Medications
- Route and dosage of medications
- Times of administration of medication

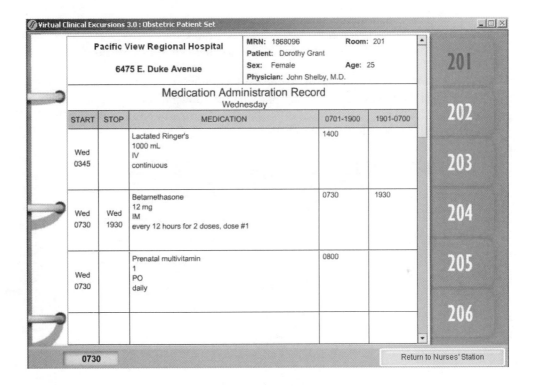

Note: The MAR changes each day. Expired MARs are stored in the patients' charts.

CHARTS

To access patient charts, either click on the **Chart** icon at the top of your screen or anywhere within the chart rack in the center of the Nurses' Station screen. When the close-up view appears, the individual charts are labeled by room number. To open a chart, click on the room number of the patient whose chart you wish to review. The patient's name and allergies will appear, along with a list of tabs on the right side of the screen, allowing you to view the following data:

- Allergies
- Physician's Orders
- Physician's Notes
- Nurse's Notes
- Laboratory Reports
- Diagnostic Reports
- Surgical Reports
- Consultations

- Patient Education
- History and Physical
- Nursing Admission
- Expired MARs
- Consents
- Mental Health
- Admissions
- Emergency Department

Information appears in real time. The entries are in reverse chronological order, so use the down arrow at the right side of the chart page to scroll down to view previous entries. Flip from tab to tab to view multiple data fields or click on the **Return to Nurses' Station** bar in the lower right corner of the screen to exit the chart.

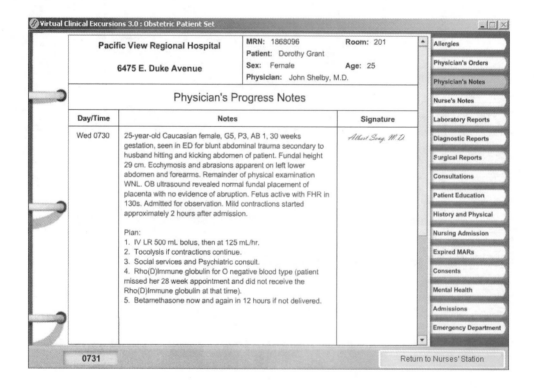

ELECTRONIC PATIENT RECORD (EPR)

The EPR can be accessed from the computer in the Nurses' Station or from the EPR icon located in the tool bar at the top of your screen. To access a patient's EPR:
- Click on either the computer screen or the **EPR** icon.
- Your user name and password are automatically filled in.
- Click on **Login** to enter the EPR.

The EPR used in Pacific View Regional Hospital represents a composite of commercial versions being used in hospitals. You can access the EPR:
- for a patient (by room number).
- to review existing data.
- to enter data you collect while working with a patient.

The EPR is updated daily, so no matter what day or part of a shift you are working, there will be a current EPR with the patient's data from the past days of the current hospital stay. This type of simulated EPR allows you to examine how data for different attributes have changed over time, as well as to examine data for all of a patient's attributes at a particular time. The EPR is fully functional (as it is in a real-life hospital). You can enter such data as blood pressure, breath sounds, and certain treatments. The EPR will not, however, allow you to enter data for a previous time period. Use the arrows at the bottom of the screen to move forward and backward in time.

At the top of the EPR screen, you can choose patients by their room numbers. In addition, you have access to 17 different categories of patient data. To change patients or data categories, click the down arrow to the right of the room number or category.

The categories of patient data in the EPR as as follows:

- Vital Signs
- Respiratory
- Cardiovascular
- Neurologic
- Gastrointestinal
- Excretory
- Musculoskeletal
- Integumentary
- Reproductive
- Psychosocial
- Wounds and Drains
- Activity
- Hygiene and Comfort
- Safety
- Nutrition
- IV
- Intake and Output

Remember, each hospital selects its own codes. The codes used in the EPR at Pacific View Regional Hospital may be different from ones you have seen in clinical rotations that have computerized patient records. Take some time to acquaint yourself with the codes. Within the Vital Signs category, click on any item in the left column (e.g., heart rate). In the far-right column, you will see a list of code meanings for the possible findings and/or descriptors for that assessment area.

You will use the codes to record the data you collect as you work with patients. Click on the box in the last time column to the right of the data and wait for the code meanings applicable to that entry to appear. Select the appropriate code to describe your assessment findings and type it in the box. (*Note:* If no cursor appears within the box, click on the box again until the blue shading disappears and the blinking cursor appears.) Once the data are typed in this box, they are entered into the patient's record for this period of care only.

To leave the EPR, click on **Exit EPR** in the bottom right corner of the screen.

■ **VISITING A PATIENT**

From the Nurses' Station, click on the room number of the patient you wish to visit in the tool bar at the bottom of your screen. Once you are inside the room, you will see a still photo of your patient in the top left corner. To verify that this is the patient you have chosen, click on the **Check Armband** icon to the right of the photo. The patient's identification data will appear. If you click on **Check Allergies** (the next icon to the right), a list of the patient's allergies (if any) will replace the photo.

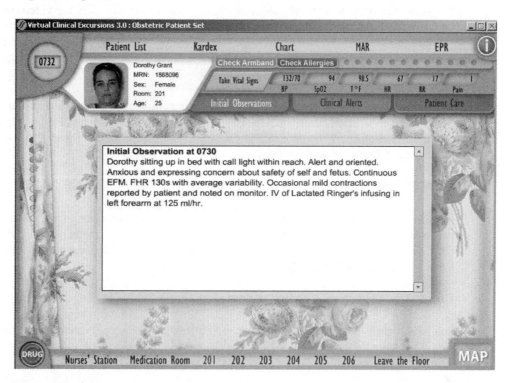

Also located in the patient's room are multiple icons you may use to assess the patient or the patient's medications. A clock is provided in the upper left corner of the room to monitor your progress in real time.

- The tool bar across the top of the screen allows you to check the **Patient List**, access the **EPR** to check or enter data, and view the patient's **Chart**, **MAR**, or **Kardex**.

- The **Take Vital Signs** icon allows you to measure the patient's up-to-the-minute blood pressure, oxygen saturation, temperature, heart rate, respiratory rate, and pain level.

- When you click on **Initial Observations**, a description appears in the text box under the patient's photo, allowing you a "look" at the patient as if you had just stepped in. To the right of this icon is **Clinical Alerts**, a resource that allows you to make decisions about priority medication interventions based on emerging data collected in real time. Check this screen throughout your period of care to avoid missing critical information related to recently ordered or STAT medications.

- Clicking on the **Patient Care** icon opens up three specific learning environments within the patient room: **Physical Assessment**, **Nurse-Client Interactions**, and **Medication Administration**.

- To perform a **Physical Assessment**, choose a body area (such as **Head & Neck**) by clicking on the appropriate icon in the column of yellow buttons. This activates a list of system subcategories for that body area (e.g., see **Sensory**, **Neurologic**, etc. in the green boxes). After you click on the system that you wish to evaluate, a still photo and text box appear, describing the assessment findings. The still photo is a "snapshot" of how an assessment of this area might be done or what the finding might look like. For every body area, there is also an **Equipment** button located on the far right of the screen.

- To the right of the Physical Assessment icon is **Nurse-Client Interactions**. Clicking on this icon will reveal the times and titles of any videos available for viewing. (*Note:* If the video you wish to see is not listed, this means you have not yet reached the correct virtual time to view that video. Check the virtual clock; you may return to access the video once its designated time has occurred—as long as you do so within the corresponding period of care.) To view a listed video, click on the white arrow to the right of the video title. Use the square control buttons below the video to start, stop, pause, rewind, or fast-forward the action or to mute the sound.

- **Medication Administration** is the pathway that allows you to review and administer medications to a patient after you have prepared them in the Medication Room. This process is addressed further in the *How to Prepare Medications* section (pages 19-20) and in *A Detailed Tour* (pages 26-30).

■ HOW TO QUIT, CHANGE PATIENTS, OR CHANGE PERIOD OF CARE

How to Quit: From most screens, you may click the **Leave the Floor** icon on the bottom tool bar to the right of the patient room numbers. (*Note:* From some screens, you will first need to click an **Exit** button or **Return to Nurses' Station** before clicking **Leave the Floor**.) When the Floor Menu appears, click **Exit** to leave the program.

How to Change Patients, Floors, or Period of Care: To change patients, simply click on the new patient's room number. (You cannot receive a scorecard for a new patient, however, unless you have already selected that patient on the Patient List screen.) To change to a new period of care, to change floors, or to restart the virtual clock for a new patient, click the **Leave the Floor** icon and then **Restart**.

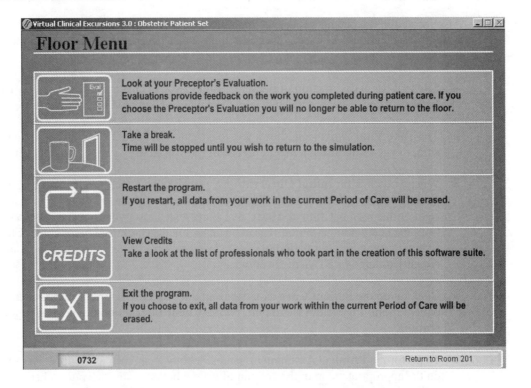

■ HOW TO PREPARE MEDICATIONS

From the Nurses' Station or the patient's room, you can access the Medication Room by clicking on the icon in the tool bar at the bottom of your screen to the left of the patient room numbers.

In the Medication Room you have access to the following (from left to right):

- A preparation area is located on the counter under the cabinets. To begin the medication preparation process, click on the tray on the counter or click on the **Preparation** icon at the top of the screen. The next screen leads you through a preparation sequence (called the Preparation Wizard) to prepare medications one at a time for administration to a patient. However, no medication has been selected at this time. We will do this while working with a patient in *A Detailed Tour*. To exit this screen, click on **View the Medication Room**.

- To the right of the cabinets (and above the refrigerator), IV storage bins are provided. Click on the bins themselves or on the **IV Storage** icon at the top of the screen. The bins are labeled **Microinfusion**, **Small Volume**, and **Large Volume**. Click on an individual bin to see a list of its contents. No medications are available in the bins at this time, but if they were, you could click on an individual medication and its label would appear to the right under the patient's name. Next, you would click **Put Medication on Tray**. If you ever change your mind or choose the incorrect medication, you can reverse your actions by clicking on **Put Medication in Bin**. Click **Close Bin** in the right bottom corner to exit. **View Medication Room** brings you back to a full view of the entire room.

- A refrigerator is located under the IV storage bins to hold any medications that must be stored below room temperature. Click on it to remove your medications; then click **Close Door**. You can also access this area by clicking the **Refrigerator** icon at the top of the screen.

- To prepare controlled substances, click the **Automated System** icon at the top of the screen or click the computer monitor located to the right of the IV storage bins. A login screen will appear; your name and password are automatically filled in. Click **Login**. Select a patient to log medications out for; then select the drawer you wish to open. Click **Open Drawer**, choose **Put Medication on Tray**, and then click **Close Drawer**.

- Next to the Automated System is a set of drawers identified by patient room number. To access these, click on the drawers themselves or on the **Unit Dosage** icon at the top of the screen. This provides a close-up view of the drawers. Click on the room number of the patient you are working with to open that drawer. Next, click on the medication you would like to prepare for the patient, and a label appears to the right under the patient's name, listing strength, units, and dosage per unit. You can **Open** and **Close** this medication label by clicking the appropriate icon. To exit, click **Close Drawer**; then click **View Medication Room**.

At any time, you can learn about a medication you wish to prepare for a patient by clicking on the **Drug** icon in the bottom left corner of the medication room screen or by clicking the **Drug Guide** book on the counter to the right of the unit dosage drawers. The **Drug Guide** provides information about the medications commonly included in nursing drug handbooks. Nutritional supplements and maintenance intravenous fluid preparations are not included.

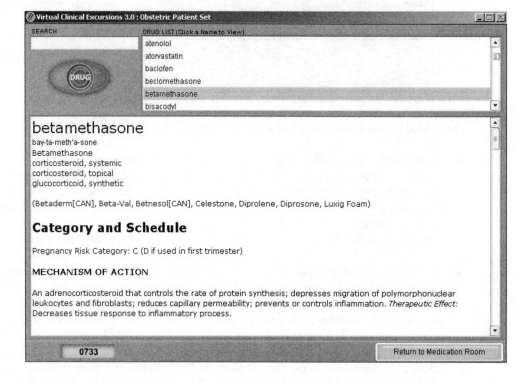

To access the MAR to review the medications ordered for a patient, click on the **MAR** icon located in the tool bar at the top of your screen. You may also click the **Review MAR** icon in the tool bar at the bottom of your screen from inside each medication storage area.

After you have chosen and prepared your medications, return to the patient's room to administer them by clicking on the room number in the bottom tool bar. Once inside the patient's room, click on **Medication Administration** and follow the administration sequence.

■ PRECEPTOR'S EVALUATIONS

When you have finished a session, click on **Leave the Floor** to go to the Floor Menu. At this point, you can click on the icon next to **Look at your Preceptor's Evaluation** to receive a scorecard that provides feedback on the work you completed during patient care.

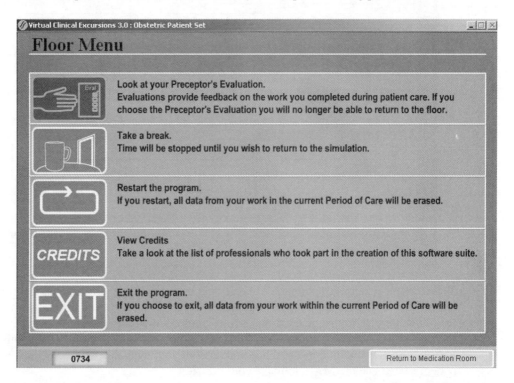

Evaluations are available for each patient you signed in for. Click on any of the **Medication Scorecard** icons to see an example. The scorecard compares the medications you administered to a patient during a period of care with what should have been administered. Table A lists the correct medications. Table B lists any medications that were administered incorrectly.

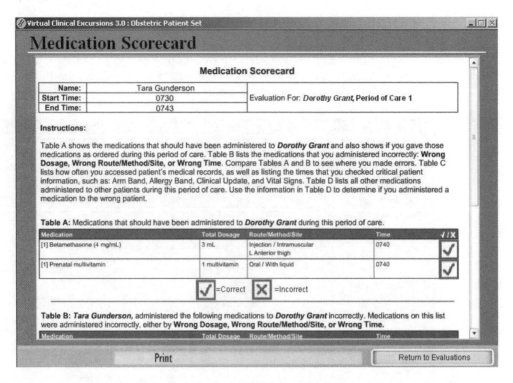

Not every medication listed on the MAR should be given. For example, a patient might have an allergy to a drug that was ordered, or a medication might have been improperly transcribed to the MAR. Predetermined medication "errors" embedded within the program challenge you to exercise critical thinking skills and professional judgment when deciding to administer a medication, just as you would in a real hospital. Use all your available resources, such as the patient's chart and the MAR, to make your decision.

Table C lists the resources that were available to assist you in medication administration, and it documents whether and when you accessed these resources. For example, did you check the patient armband or perform a check of vital signs? If so, when?

You can click **Print** to get a copy of this report if needed. Click **Return to Evaluations** when finished.

■ FLOOR MAP

To get a general sense of your location within the hospital, click on the **Map** icon found in the lower right corner of most of the screens in the *Virtual Clinical Excursions—Obstetrics* program. A floor map will appear, showing the layout of the floor you are currently on, as well as a directory of the patients and services on that floor. As you move your cursor over the directory list, the location of each room is highlighted (and vice versa). The floor map can be accessed from the Nurses' Station, Medication Room, and each patient's room.

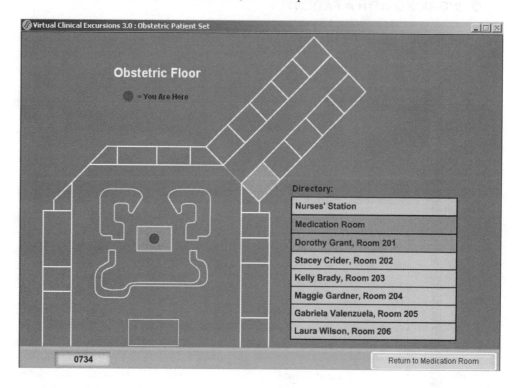

A DETAILED TOUR

If you wish to more thoroughly understand the capabilities of *Virtual Clinical Excursions—Obstetrics*, take a detailed tour by completing the following section. During this tour, we will work with a specific patient to introduce you to all the different components and learning opportunities available within the software.

■ WORKING WITH A PATIENT

Sign in to work on the Obstetrics Floor for Period of Care 1 (0730-0815). From the Patient List, select Dorothy Grant in Room 201; however, do not go to the Nurses' Station yet.

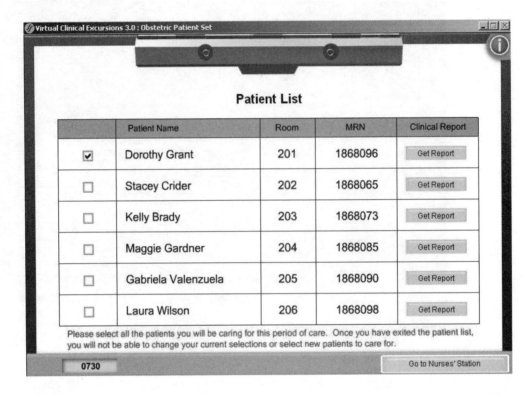

■ REPORT

In hospitals, when one shift ends and another begins, the outgoing nurse who attended a patient will give a verbal and sometimes a written summary of that patient's condition to the incoming nurse who will assume care for the patient. This summary is called a report and is an important source of data to provide an overview of a patient. Your first task is to get clinical report on Dorothy Grant. To do this, click **Get Report** in the far right column in this patient's row. From this summary, identify the problems and areas of concern that you will need to address for this patient.

When you have finished reading the report and noting any areas of concern, click **Go to Nurses' Station**.

■ CHARTS

You can access Dorothy Grant's chart from the Nurses' Station or from the patient's room (201). We will access it from the Nurses' Station: Click on the chart rack or on the **Chart** icon in the tool bar at the top of your screen. Next, click on the chart labeled **201** to open the medical record for Dorothy Grant. Click on the **Emergency Department** tab to view a record of why this patient was admitted.

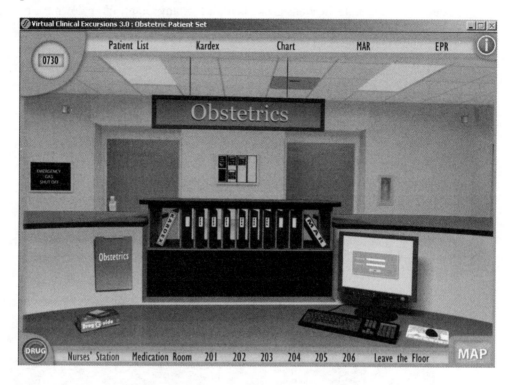

How many days has Dorothy Grant been in the hospital?

What tests were done upon her arrival in the Emergency Department and why?

What was the reason for her admission?

You should also click on **Surgical Reports** to learn whether any procedures were performed and when. Finally, review the **Nursing Admission** and **History and Physical** tabs to view information on the health history of this patient. When you are done reviewing the chart, click **Return to Nurses' Station**.

■ MEDICATIONS

Open the Medication Administration Record (MAR) by clicking on the **MAR** icon in the tool bar at the top of your screen. *Remember:* The MAR automatically opens to the first occupied room number on the floor. Since you need to access Dorothy Grant's MAR, click on tab **201** (her room number). Always make sure you are giving the *Right Drug to the Right Patient!*

Examine the list of medications prescribed for Dorothy Grant. Write down the medications that need to be given during this period of care (0730-0815). For each medication, note the dosage, route, and time in the chart below.

Time	Medication	Dosage	Route

Click on **Return to Nurses' Station**. Next, click on **201** on the bottom tool bar and then verify that you are indeed in Dorothy Grant's room. Select **Clinical Alerts** (the icon to the right of Initial Observations) to check for any emerging data that might affect your medication administration priorities. Go to the patient's chart (click on the **Chart** icon; then click on **201**). When the chart opens, select the **Physician's Orders** tab.

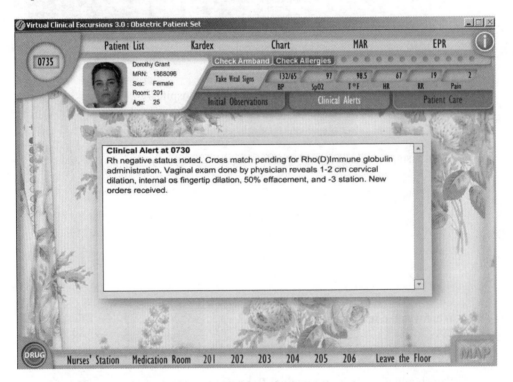

Review the orders. Have any new medications been ordered? Return to the MAR (click **Return to Room 201**; then click **MAR**). Verify that the new medications have been correctly transcribed to the MAR. Mistakes are sometimes made in the transcription process in the hospital setting, and it is sound practice to double-check any new order.

Are there any patient assessments you will need to perform before administering these medications? If so, return to Room 201 and click on **Review of Systems** to complete those before proceeding.

Now click on the **Medication Room** icon in the tool bar at the bottom of your screen to locate and prepare the medications for Dorothy Grant.

In the Medication Room, you must access the medications for Dorothy Grant from the specific dispensing system in which each medication is stored. Locate each medication that needs to be given in this time period and click on **Put Medication on Tray** as appropriate. (*Hint:* Look in Unit Dosage drawer first.) When you are finished, click on **Close Drawer** and then on **View Medication Room**. Now click on the medication tray on the counter on the left side of the medication room screen to begin preparing the medications you have selected. (*Note:* Instead of clicking on the tray, you can click **Preparation** at top of screen.)

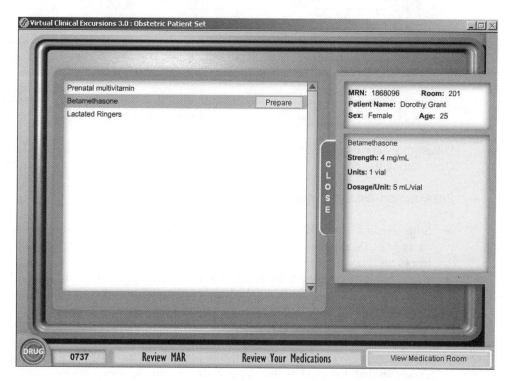

In the preparation area, you should see a list of the medications you put on the tray in the previous steps. Click on the first medication and then click **Prepare**. Follow the onscreen instructions of the Preparation Wizard, providing any data requested. As an example, let's follow the preparation process for betamethasone, one of the medications due to be administered to Dorothy Grant during this period of care. To begin, click on **Betamethasone**; then click **Prepare**. Now work through the Preparation Wizard sequence as detailed below:

Amount of medication in the ampule: 5 mL
Enter the amount of medication you will draw up into a syringe: **3** mL
Click **Next**.
Select the patient you wish to set aside the medication for:
Click **Room 201, Dorothy Grant**.
Click **Finish**.
Click **Return to Medication Room**.

Follow this same basic process for the other medications due to be administered to Dorothy Grant during this period of care. (*Hint:* Look in **IV Storage** and **Automated System**.)

PREPARATION WIZARD EXCEPTIONS

- Some medications in *Virtual Clinical Excursions—Obstetrics* are preprepared by the pharmacy (e.g., IV antibiotics) and taken to the patient room as a whole. This is common practice in most hospitals.
- Blood products are not administered by students through the *Virtual Clinical Excursions—Obstetrics* simulations since blood administration follows specific protocols not covered in this program.
- The *Virtual Clinical Excursions—Obstetrics* simulations do not allow for mixing more than one type of medication, such as regular and Lente insulins, in the same syringe. In the clinical setting, when multiple types of insulin are ordered for a patient, the regular insulin is drawn up first, followed by the longer-acting insulin. Insulin is always administered in a special unit-marked syringe.

Now return to Room 201 (click on **201** on bottom tool bar) to administer Dorothy Grant's medications.

At any time during the medication administration process, you can perform a further review of systems, take vital signs, check information contained within the chart, or verify patient identity and allergies. Inside Dorothy Grant's room, click **Take Vital Signs**. (*Note:* These findings change over time to reflect the temporal changes you would find in a patient similar to Dorothy Grant.)

When you have gathered all the data you need, click on **Patient Care** and then select **Medication Administration**. After reviewing your medications, continue the administration process with the betamethasone ordered for Dorothy Grant. In the list of medications set aside for this patient, click to highlight **Betamethasone**. Next, click on the down arrow to the right of **Select** and choose **Administer** from the drop-down menu. This will activate the Administration Wizard. Complete the Wizard sequence as follows:

- Route: **Injection**
- Method: **Intramuscular**
- Site: **Any**
- Click **Administer to Patient** arrow.
- Would you like to document this administration in the MAR? **Yes**
- Click **Finish** arrow.

Selections are recorded by a tracking system and evaluated on a Medication Scorecard stored under Preceptor's Evaluations. This scorecard can be viewed, printed, and given to your instructor. To access the Preceptor's Evaluations, click on **Leave the Floor**. When the Floor Menu appears, click on the icon next to **Look at Your Preceptor's Evaluation**. From the list of evaluations, click on **Medication Scorecard** inside the box with Dorothy Grant's name.

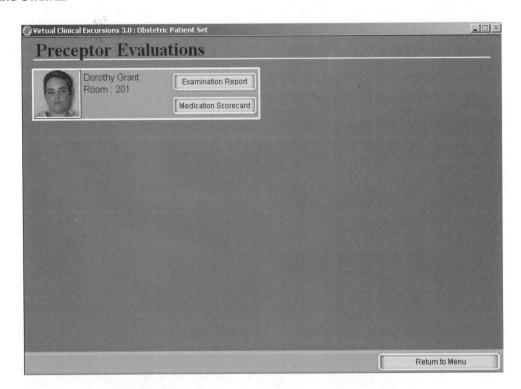

■ MEDICATION SCORECARD

- First, review Table A. Was betamethasone given correctly? Did you give the other medications as ordered?
- Table B shows you which (if any) medications you gave incorrectly.
- Table C addresses the resources used for Dorothy Grant. Did you access the patient's chart, MAR, EPR, or Kardex as needed to make safe medication administration decisions?
- Did you check the patient's armband to verify her identity? Did you check whether your patient had any known allergies to medications? Were vital signs taken?

■ VITAL SIGNS

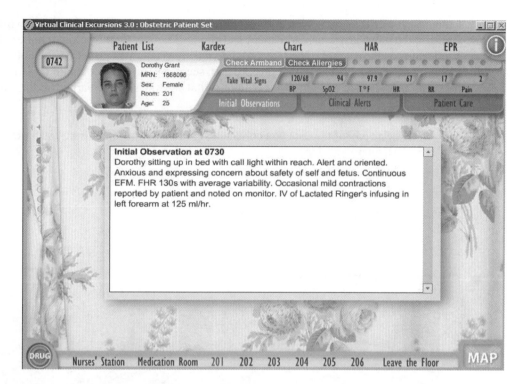

Vital signs, often considered the traditional signs of life, include body temperature, heart rate, respiratory rate, blood pressure, oxygen saturation of the blood, and the patient's experience of pain.

Inside Dorothy Grant's room, click **Take Vital Signs**. (*Remember:* You can take vital signs at any time. The data change over time to reflect the temporal changes you would find in a patient similar to Dorothy Grant.) Collect vital signs for this patient and record them in the following table. Note the time at which you collected each of these data.

Vital Signs	Findings/Time
Blood pressure	
O$_2$ saturation	
Heart rate	
Respiratory rate	
Temperature	
Pain rating	

After you are done, click on the **EPR** icon located in the tool bar at the top of the screen.

Complete the EPR Login screen as directed in *A Quick Tour* (see page 15 of this workbook). Click on the down arrow next to Patient and choose Dorothy Grant's room number **201**. Select **Vital Signs** as the category. Next, record the vital signs data you just collected in the last column. (*Note:* If you need help with this process, see page 16.) Now compare these findings with the data you collected earlier for this patient's vital signs. Use these earlier findings to establish a baseline for each of the vital signs.

> a. Are any of the data you collected significantly different from the baseline for a particular vital sign?
>
> Circle One: Yes   No
>
> b. If "Yes," which data are different?

■ PHYSICAL ASSESSMENT

After you have finished examining the EPR for vital signs, click **Exit EPR** to return to Room 201. Click **Patient Care** and then **Physical Assessment**. Think about what information you received in report, as well as what you may have learned about this patient from the chart. What area(s) of examination should you pay most attention to at this time? Is there any equipment you should be monitoring? Conduct a physical assessment of the body areas and systems that you consider priorities for Dorothy Grant. For example, select **Head & Neck**; then click on and assess **Mental Status** and **Equipment**. Complete any other assessment(s) you think are necessary at this time. In the following table, record the data you collected during this examination.

Area of Examination	Findings
Head & Neck Mental Status	
Head & Neck Equipment	

After you have finished collecting these data, return to the EPR. Compare the data that were already in the record with those you just collected.

a. Are any of the data you collected significantly different from the baselines for this patient?

Circle One: Yes   No

b. If "Yes," which data are different?

■ NURSE-CLIENT INTERACTIONS

Click on **Patient Care** from inside Dorothy Grant's room (201). Now click on **Nurse-Client Interactions** to access a short video titled **Patient Teaching—Medication**, which is available for viewing at 0730 (based on the virtual clock in the upper left corner of your screen). To begin the video, click on the arrow next to its title. You will observe a nurse communicating with Dorothy Grant. There are many variations of nursing practice, some exemplifying "best" practice and some not. Note whether the nurse in this interaction displays professional behavior and compassionate care. Are her words congruent with what is going on with the patient? Does this interaction "feel right" to you? If not, how would you handle this situation differently? Explain.

Note: If the video you wish to view is not listed, this means you have not yet reached the correct virtual time to view that video. Check the virtual clock; you may return to access the video once its designated time has occurred—as long as you do so within the corresponding period of care.

At least one Nurse-Client Interactions video is available during each period of care. Viewing these videos can help you learn more about what is occurring with a patient at a certain time and also prompt you to discriminate between nurse communications that are ideal and those that need improvement. Compassionate care and the ability to communicate clearly are essential components of delivering quality nursing care, and it is during your clinical time that you will begin to refine these skills.

■ COLLECTING AND EVALUATING DATA

Each of the activities you perform in the Patient Care environment generates a great deal of assessment data. Remember that after you collect data, you can record your findings in the EPR. You can also review the EPR, patient's chart, videos, and MAR at any time. You will get plenty of practice collecting and then evaluating data in context of the patient's course.

Now, here's an important question for you:

> Did the previous sequence of exercises provide the most efficient way to assess Dorothy Grant?

For example, you went to the patient's room to get vital signs, then back to the EPR to enter data and compare your findings with extant data. Next, you went back to the patient's room to do a physical examination, then again back to the EPR to enter and review data. If this back-and-forth process of data collection and recording seemed inefficient, remember the following:

- Plan all of your nursing activities to maximize efficiency while at the same time optimizing quality of patient care. (Think about what data you might need to perform certain tasks. For example, do you need to check a heart rate before administering a cardiac medication or check an IV site before starting an infusion?)

- You collect a tremendous amount of data when you work with a patient. Very few people can accurately remember all these data for more than a few minutes. Develop efficient assessment skills, and record data as soon as possible after collecting them.

- Assessment data are only the starting point for the nursing process.

Make a clear distinction between these first exercises and how you actually provide nursing care. These initial exercises were designed to involve you actively in the use of different software components. This workbook focuses on sensible practices for implementing the nursing process in ways that ensure the highest quality care of patients.

Most important, remember that a human being changes through time, and that these changes include both the physical and psychosocial facets of a person as a living organism. Think about this for a moment. Some patients may change physically in a very short time (a patient with emerging myocardial infarction) or more slowly (a patient with a chronic illness). Patients' overall physical and psychosocial conditions may improve or deteriorate. They may have effective coping skills and familial support, or they may feel alone and full of despair. In fact, each individual is a complex mix of physical and psychosocial elements, and at least some of these elements usually change through time.

Thus it is crucial *not* to think of the nursing process as a simple one-time, five-step procedure:

- Assessment
- Nursing Diagnosis
- Planning
- Implementation
- Evaluation

Rather, the nursing process should be utilized as a creative and systematic approach to delivering nursing care. Furthermore, because all living organisms are constantly changing, we must apply the nursing process over and over. Each time we follow the nursing process for an individual patient, we refine our understanding of that patient's physical and psychosocial conditions based on collection and analysis of many different types of data. *Virtual Clinical Excursions—Obstetrics* will help you develop both the creativity and the systematic approach needed to become a nurse who is equipped to deliver the highest quality care to all patients.

■ REDUCING MEDICATION ERRORS: SELF-EVALUATION

Earlier in this detailed tour, you learned the basic steps of medication preparation and administration. The following simulations will allow you to practice those skills further—with an increased emphasis on reducing medication errors by using the Medication Scorecard to evaluate your work.

Sign in to work at Pacific View Regional Hospital for Period of Care 1. (*Note:* If you are already working with another patient or during another period of care, click on **Leave the Floor** and then **Restart the Program**; then sign in.)

From the Patient List, select Dorothy Grant. Then click on **Go to Nurses' Station**. Complete the following steps to prepare and administer medications to Dorothy Grant.

- Click on **Medication Room**.
- Click on **MAR** to determine prn medications that have been ordered for Dorothy Grant. (*Note:* You may click on **Review MAR** at any time to verify correct medication order. Remember to look at the patient name on the MAR to make sure you have the correct patient's record—you must click on the correct room number within the MAR.) Click on **Return to Medication Room** after reviewing the correct MAR.
- Click on **Unit Dosage** (or on the Unit Dosage cabinet); from the close-up view, click on drawer **201**.
- Select the medications you would like to administer. After each selection, click **Put Medication on Tray**. When you are finished selecting medications, click **Close Drawer**.
- Click on **View Medication Room**.
- Click on **Automated System** (or on the Automated System unit itself). Click **Login**.
- On the next screen, specify the correct patient and drawer location.
- Select the medication you would like to administer and click on **Put Medication on Tray**. Repeat this process if you wish to administer other medications from the Automated System.
- When you are finished, click **Close Drawer**. At the bottom right corner of the next screen, click on **View Medication Room**.
- From the Medication Room, click on **Preparation** (or on the preparation tray).
- From the list of medications on your tray, choose the correct medication to administer.
- Click **Next**, specify the correct patient to administer this medication to, and click **Finish**.
- Repeat the previous two steps until all medications that you want to administer are prepared.
- You can click on **Review Your Medications** and then on **Return to Medication Room** when ready. Once you are back in the Medication Room, go directly to Dorothy Grant's room by clicking on **201** at bottom of screen.
- Inside the patient's room, administer the medication, utilizing the five rights of medication administration. After you have collected the appropriate assessment data and are ready for administration, click **Patient Care** and then **Medication Administration**. Verify that the correct patient and medication(s) appear in the left-hand window. Then click the down arrow next to Select. From the drop-down menu, select **Administer** and complete the Administration Wizard by providing any information requested. When the Wizard stops asking for information, click **Administer to Patient**. Specify **Yes** when asked whether this administration should be recorded in the MAR. Finally, click **Finish**.

Now let's see how you did during your earlier medication administration!

- Click on **Leave the Floor** at the bottom of your screen. From the Floor Menu, select **Look at Your Preceptor's Evaluation**. Then click on **Medication Scorecard**.

These resources will help you find out more about each patient's medications and possible sources of medication errors.

1. Start by examining Table A. These are the medications you should have given to Dorothy Grant during this period of care. If each of the medications in Table A has a ✓ by it, then you made no errors. Congratulations!

If there are some medications that have an X by them, then you made one or more medication errors.

Compare Tables A and B to determine which of the following types of errors you made: Wrong Dose, Wrong Route/Method/Site, or Wrong Time. Follow these steps:
   a. Find medications in Table A that were given incorrectly.
   b. Now see if those same medications are in Table B, which shows what you actually administered to Dorothy Grant.
   c. Comparing Tables A and B, match the Strength, Dose, Route/Method/Site, and Time for each medication you administered incorrectly.
   d. Then, using the form below, list the medications given incorrectly and mark the errors you made for each medication.

Medication	Strength	Dosage	Route	Method	Site	Time
	❏	❏	❏	❏	❏	❏
	❏	❏	❏	❏	❏	❏
	❏	❏	❏	❏	❏	❏
	❏	❏	❏	❏	❏	❏

2. To help you reduce future medication errors, consider the following list of possible reasons for errors.

   • Did not check drug against MAR for correct patient, correct date, correct time, correct drug, and correct dose.
   • Did not check drug dose against MAR three times.
   • Did not open the unit dose package in the patient's room.
   • Did not correctly identify the patient using two identifiers.
   • Did not administer the drug on time.
   • Did not verify patient allergies.
   • Did not check the patient's current condition or vital sign parameters.
   • Did not consider why the patient would be receiving this drug.
   • Did not question why the drug was in the patient's drawer.
   • Did not check the physician's order and/or check with the pharmacist when there was a question about the drug or dose.
   • Did not verify that no adverse effects had occurred from a previous dose.

Based on these possibilities, determine how you made each error and record the reason into the form below:

Medication	Reason for Error

3. Look again at Table B. Are there medications listed that are not in Table A? If so, you gave a medication to Dorothy Grant that he should not have received. Complete the following exercises to help you understand how such an error might have been made.

   a. Perhaps you gave a medication that was on Dorothy Grant's MAR for this period of care, without recognizing that a change had occurred in the patient's condition that should have caused you to reconsider. Review patient records as necessary and complete the following form:

Medication	Possible Reasons Not to Give This Medication

   b. Another possibility is that you gave Dorothy Grant a medication that should have been given at a different time. Check his MAR and complete the form below to determine whether you made a Wrong Time error:

Medication	Given to Dorothy Grant at What Time	Should Have Been Given at What Time

c. Maybe you gave another patient's medication to Dorothy Grant. In this case, you made a Wrong Patient error. Check the MARs of other patients and use the form below to determine whether you made this type of error:

Medication	Given to Dorothy Grant	Should Have Been Given to

4. The Medication Scorecard provides some other interesting sources of information. For example, if there is a medication selected for Dorothy Grant but it was not given to him, there will be an X by that medication in Table A, but it will not appear in Table B. In that case, you might have given this medication to some other patient, which is another type of Wrong Patient error. To investigate further, look at Table D, which lists the medications you gave to other patients. See whether you can find any medications for Dorothy Grant that were given to another patient by mistake. Before making any decisions, be sure to cross-check the other patients' MAR because they may have had the same medication ordered. Use the following form to record your findings:

Medication	Should Have Been Given to Dorothy Grant	Given by Mistake to

5. Now take some time to review the exercises you just completed. Use the form below to create an overall analysis of what you have learned. Once again, record each of the medication errors you made, including the type of each error. Then, for each error you made, indicate specifically what you would do differently to prevent this type of error from occurring again.

Medication	Type of Error	Error Prevention Tactic

Submit this form to your instructor if required as a graded assignment, or simply use these exercises to improve your understanding of medication errors and how to reduce them.

Name: _____   Date: _____

The following icons are used throughout the workbook to help you quickly identify particular activities and assignments:

 Indicates a reading assignment—tells you which textbook chapter(s) you should read before starting each lesson

 Indicates a writing activity

 Marks the beginning of an interactive CD-ROM activity—signals you to open or return to your *Virtual Clinical Excursions—Obstetrics* CD-ROM

 Indicates additional CD-ROM instructions

Indicates questions and activities that require you to consult your textbook

Indicates the approximate time required to complete an exercise

Done
on: 9/18/06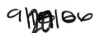

LESSON 1

Community Care: The Family and Culture

 Reading Assignment: Community Care: The Family and Culture (Chapter 2)

Patients: Dorothy Grant, Room 201
Stacey Crider, Room 202
Kelly Brady, Room 203
Maggie Gardner, Room 204
Gabriela Valenzuela, Room 205
Laura Wilson, Room 206

Goal: Demonstrate an understanding of how the family, community, and culture affects the pregnant women.

Objectives:

- Discuss the various types of families, communities, and cultures represented by each of the patients.
- Assess and plan care for a patient from a specific culture.
- Explore how your background influences the care that you give to patients who have differing experiences in regard to community, family, or culture.

Exercise 1

 CD-ROM Activity

15 minutes

Review pages 18-19 of Chapter 2 in your textbook and complete the following exercise regarding family types.

Read question 1 before starting this period of care. Fill in the table as you review each patient's chart.

- Sign in to work at Pacific View Regional Hospital on the Obstetrics Floor for Period of Care 1. (*Note*: If you are already in the virtual hospital from a previous exercise, click on **Leave the Floor** and then **Restart the Program** to get to the sign-in window.)

- From the Patient List, select all six patients.
- Click on **Go to Nurses' Station** and then on **Chart**.
- Click on Dorothy Grant's chart (**201**) to begin.
- Click on the **Admissions** tab and find the patient's marital status.
- Click on the **History and Physical** tab and review the Family History section.
- Once you have completed the column for Dorothy Grant in the table below, click on **Return to Nurses' Station** and review Stacey Crider's chart (**202**). Repeat this sequence until you have completed question 1.

1. Under each patient's name below, place an X to indicate that patient's type of family.

	Dorothy Grant	Stacey Crider	Kelly Brady	Maggie Gardner	Gabriela Valenzuela	Laura Wilson
Nuclear	X	X	X	X	X	X
Binuclear						
Extended		X	X			
Single-parent				X		X
Blended						

2. Using what you learned in your chart review combined with the information in your textbook, describe the type of family that Gabriela Valenzuela has.

Gabriella has a nuclear family b/c she's living w/ her husband although his family is supportive, it doesn't state they all live in the same house.

3. Based on the information provided in your textbook, what type of family do you have? Describe how your family fits the description of the family type that you have chosen.

nuclear family

Exercise 2

 CD-ROM Activity

 15 minutes

Just as there are different types of families, there are also various populations of women within every community. To gain a better understanding of this, read pages 23-25 of the textbook.

Read question 1 before starting this period of care. Fill in the table as you review each patient's chart.

- Sign in to work at Pacific View Regional Hospital on the Obstetrics Floor for Period of Care 1. (*Note*: If you are already in the virtual hospital from a previous exercise, click on Leave the Floor and then **Restart the Program** to get to the sign-in window.)
- From the Patient List, select all six patients.
- Click on **Go to Nurses' Station** and then on **Chart**.
- Select Dorothy Grant's chart (**201**) to begin.
- Click on the **Nursing Admissions** tab. (*Hint*: The first four pages of this section will provide information regarding patient's population.)
- You may also click on the **History and Physical** for information to complete the table below.
- Once you have completed Dorothy Grant's column in question 1, click on **Return to Nurses' Station**. Repeat the above steps for each patient.

1. Under each patient's name in the table below, place an X next to each description that applies.

	Dorothy Grant	Stacey Crider	Kelly Brady	Maggie Gardner	Gabriela Valenzuela	Laura Wilson
Adolescent						X
Minority		X			X	
Older			X	X		
Incarcerated						
Migrant						
Homeless	X					
Immigrant					X	

2. Laura Wilson is a member of one of the most medically underserved groups. What are two lifestyle choices she has made that represent high-risk behaviors common in this group?

DRUG ABUSE & SEXUALLY ACTIVE

3. According to information in your textbook, Dorothy Grant could be classified as homeless. What are two contributing factors seen in homeless women?

DOMESTIC VIOLENCE & not employed

4. According to the textbook, older pregnant women, such as Maggie Gardner, are less likely to use *preventive* services, leading to *chronic illnesses*.

5. According to the textbook, minority women with underlying health conditions have an increased risk for *poor obstetric outcomes for themselves & infants*.

6. What has your experience been with caring for these types of patients?

I realize that I will interact w/ many different types of patients, and I should treat each of them with the same type of respect. Moreover, not all patients will come in w/ the same type of problems or situations, so each must be cared for with the same type of respect but different tactics.

7. Based on the information found in the textbook, will you change the way you care for these types of patients in the future? If so, how? In your community, what resources are available for women who are affected by the issues discussed in this exercise?

 Exercise 3

 CD-ROM Activity

25 minutes

- Sign in to work at Pacific View Regional Hospital on the Obstetrics Floor for Period of Care 1. (*Note*: If you are already in the virtual hospital from a previous exercise, click on **Leave the Floor** and then **Restart the Program** to get to the sign-in window.)
- From the Patient List, select Stacey Crider and Maggie Gardner.
- Click on **Go to Nurses' Station**.

- Click on **Chart** and then on **202**.
- Click on the **Nursing Admission** tab.
- Review Stacey Crider's Nursing Admission. (*Hint*: See the Role Relationships section.)

they have a hard situation →

1. Identify a nursing diagnosis that would be appropriate for Stacey Crider and her family.

HUSBAND SHOULD TRY TO FIND MORE RELIABLE JOB. & get papers in

- Now, click on **Return to Nurses' Station** and open Maggie Gardner's chart by clicking on **Chart** and then on **204**.
- Click on the **Nursing Admission** tab.
- Review Maggie Gardner's Nursing Admission (*Hint*: See the Health Promotion section.)

2. What alternative therapy/complementary therapy does Maggie Gardner use to relieve stomach trouble?

well b/c Mrs. Gardner has high anxiety she should relax

Cascara Sagrada any time Stomach bothers Lee

3. According to the chart on page 30 in the textbook, what other condition(s) do members of Maggie Gardner's cultural group tend to self-treat during pregnancy?

AA self-treat for the discomforts of pregnancy ex. nausea vomiting constipation headache & heartburn

Maggie Gardner and her husband are very religious. According to the textbook, most members of the African-American culture have strong feelings about family, community, and religion. With this information in mind, complete the following activity and questions.

- Click on **Return to Nurses' Station**.
- Click on Room **204** at the bottom of the screen.
- Click on **Patient Care**.
- Click on **Nurse-Client Interactions**.
- Select and view the video titled **0730: Communicating Empathy**. (*Note*: If this video is not available, check the virtual clock to see whether enough time has elapsed. The video cannot be viewed before its specified time.)

4. What does Maggie Gardner's husband verbalize during this interaction that would correlate with the African-American population's deep sense of religion?

5. Based on interacting with patients in the hospital where you have worked, describe your experience(s) with caring for someone of a different culture. What are some of the ideals that are different from your own? What barriers have you experienced to your care?

6. How comfortable are you with caring for patients from a different culture? Do you find yourself feeling judgmental or attempting to change others? What can you do to learn more about other cultures?

7. What resources are available at your hospital or within your community to enhance your ability to care for a culturally diverse population?

To further explore Jim and Maggie Gardner's spiritual perspective of this event, return to the patient's chart.

→ • Click on **Chart** and then on **204**.
 • Click on the **Consultations** tab.
 • Review the Pastoral Care Spiritual Assessment and the Pastoral Consultation. (*Hint:* Be sure to scroll down to read all the pages in this section.)

8. What does Maggie Gardner "blame" her miscarriages on?

her harsh feelings toward her sister

9. Based on your review, what is Maggie Gardner's perception of God?

punishing her for something she's done

10. Based on your review of Maggie Gardner's chart during this exercise, what is one underlying theme that you see in the Consultations, Nursing Admission, and History and Physical in regard to religion and this patient's perception of her situation?

It all lies in the hands of God. He will decide whether or not she is 'good' enough for a healthy baby

Assessment and Health Promotion

📖 **Reading Assignment:** Assessment and Health Promotion (Chapter 5)

Patients: Maggie Gardner, Room 204
Laura Wilson, Room 206
Gabriela Valenzuela, Room 205

Goal: To identify the variations found in a pregnant patient's assessment, including health risk behaviors and health promotion techniques to assist in the optimal outcome for the fetus.

Objectives:

- Discuss the variations in a pregnant patient's assessment findings.
- Identify health risks in pregnant patients.
- Explore health promotion interventions that can and should be completed by the nurse caring for those patients with high-risk behaviors.

Exercise 1

 CD-ROM Activity

 20 minutes

 Review pages 94-100 in your textbook to answer the questions in this exercise.

1. According to the textbook, what are the normal findings for a breast assessment?

- Sign in to work at Pacific View Regional Hospital on the Obstetrics Floor for Period of Care 1. (*Note*: If you are already in the virtual hospital from a previous exercise, click on **Leave the Floor** and then **Restart the Program** to get to the sign-in window.)
- From the Patient List, select Maggie Gardner.
- Click on **Go to Nurses' Station**.
- Go to the patient's room by clicking on **204** at the bottom of the screen.
- Click on the **Patient Care** icon.
- Click on **Chest** in the vertical row of yellow buttons.
- Click on the green button labeled **Breasts**. Observe the breast assessment.

2. Compare and contrast the normal breast assessment findings described in the textbook with Maggie Gardner's findings.

- Still in Maggie Gardner's room, click on **Chart** at the top of the screen.
- Click on chart **204**.
- Click on the **Nursing Admission** tab and review question 13 on page 5.

3. As a part of health promotion for this patient, complete the following:

a. Does Maggie Gardner do monthly breast self-exams?

b. Has she ever had a mammogram?

c. According to the textbook, what is the recommendation regarding mammograms in Maggie Gardner's age group? (*Hint*: See page 127.)

d. Based on your textbook reading, what should Maggie Gardner be taught about breast self-examination?

- According to the textbook, there are many barriers to seeking health care. We see this is true with Maggie Gardner also. Continue reviewing the Nursing Admission section of her chart to answer the following questions regarding these barriers.

4. What are three barriers, identified in Chapter 5 of the textbook, to seeking health care?

5. Maggie Gardner, in her interaction with the nurse, identifies the barrier that prevented her from seeking heath care. What was this barrier?

Exercise 2

CD-ROM Activity

 40 minutes

- Sign in to work at Pacific View Regional Hospital on the Obstetrics Floor for Period of Care 3. (*Note*: If you are already in the virtual hospital from a previous exercise, click on **Leave the Floor** and then **Restart the Program** to get to the sign-in window.)
- From the Patient List, select Laura Wilson.
- Click on **Go to Nurses' Station**.
- Click on **Chart** and then on **206**.
- Review the **History and Physical** and the **Nursing Admission** to obtain the following information.

Along with barriers to getting health care, specific health risks occur during the childbearing years. In this exercise, we will consider these risks in relation to Laura Wilson in Room 206.

1. List the areas that put Laura Wilson at risk during her pregnancy.

2. In the Nursing Admission form, what does Laura Wilson verbalize about her use of drugs, tobacco, and alcohol in regard to her pregnancy and outcomes for her baby?

• Click on **Return to Nurses' Station**.
 • Click on **206** at the bottom of the screen.
 • Inside the patient's room, click on **Patient Care**.
 • Click on **Nurse-Client Interactions**.
 • Select and view the video titled **1530: Discharge Planning**. (*Note:* If this video is not available, check the virtual clock to see whether enough time has elapsed. The video cannot be viewed before its specified time.)
 • After viewing the video, click on **Leave the Floor**.
 • Click on **Restart the Program**.
 • Sign in again to work at Pacific View Regional Hospital on the Obstetrics Floor, this time for Period of Care 4.
 • From the nurses' station, click on **Chart** and then on **206**.
 • Click on the **Consultations** tab and review the Psychiatric Consult.
 • Next, click on **Nurses' Notes** and review.

Answer the following questions regarding your impression of the 1530 video interaction and your chart review.

3. What was the clinician's perspective of Laura Wilson as it relates to her current life situation?

4. What was your impression of Laura Wilson?

5. What does Laura Wilson say that indicates she may not understand HIV or is in denial that it is truly a medical concern?

6. From your review of the 1530 video and the Psychiatric Consult notes, what areas of health education (health promotion) need to be the focus for Laura Wilson?

Exercise 3

  CD-ROM Activity

20 minutes

The head-to-toe assessment is a key part of obtaining data, both subjective and objective, from our patients. The following exercise will walk you through a head-to-toe assessment on a pregnant patient. The goal of this exercise is to identify those areas that are abnormal or to recognize any pregnancy-related changes in each of the body systems.

- Sign in to work at Pacific View Regional Hospital on the Obstetrics Floor for Period of Care 2. (*Note:* If you are already in the virtual hospital from a previous exercise, click on **Leave the Floor** and then **Restart the Program** to get to the sign-in window.)
- From the Patient List, select Gabriela Valenzuela.
- Click on **Go to Nurses' Station** and then on **205** at the bottom of the screen.
- Click on **Patient Care**.
- Begin your assessment by clicking on **Head & Neck** (from the list of yellow buttons) and then selecting each of the system subcategories (the green buttons) to obtain the findings for that area. Continue clicking on the yellow and green buttons as you record your findings in question 1.

1. Below and on the next page, record any abnormal findings or any changes related to pregnancy from your head-to-toe assessment of Gabriela Valenzuela.

   a. Head & Neck

   b. Chest

   c. Back & Spine

   d. Upper Extremities

   e. Abdomen

   f. Pelvic

   g. Lower Extremities

To answer the following questions, please review pages 123-127 of the textbook.

2. Once the health assessment is complete, what is the nurse's responsibility to the patient on return visits?

3. List five areas in which a nurse needs to educate women to help them maintain a healthy life.

4. Pelvic exams are recommended _____ until women are _____ years old. They

   are to be started when a female _____.

5. Holli, a 65-year-old, comes to you and states that she hates going to doctors because they always seemed to be males, but that she needs to have a physical because it has been "years." Based on your reading, how could you help Holli overcome the barriers that she has? Also, what information could you provide that would help her be prepared for the examination?

LESSON **3**

Violence Against Women

 Reading Assignment: Violence Against Women (Chapter 6)

Patient: Dorothy Grant, Room 201

Goal: To identify patients at risk for intimate partner violence, interventions to assist those at risk, and ways to educate and empower those individuals toward healthy relationships.

Objectives:

- Discuss the statistics related to intimate partner violence (IPV).
- List characteristics of battered women.
- Explore the myths and facts regarding IPV.
- Identify the nurse's role in regards to the battered woman or those affected by IPV.

In this lesson you will explore the nurse's role in intimate partner violence and the battered patient.

Exercise 1

Writing Activity

 15 minutes

To answer questions 1 through 7, review the information on pages 131-135 of the textbook.

1. Match the statistics on the right to the descriptions of abuse on the left.

   ___e___ Percentage of men who are victims
   of IPV

   ___c___ Percentage of women who are
   victims of IPV

   ___D___ Percentage of women who are
   being forced into sexual activities

   ___B___ Number of women murdered per
   day as a result of IPV

   ___f___ Estimated number of women who
   are victims of IPV annually

   ___a___ Percentage of individuals who were
   abused as children and then became abusers

   ___A___ Goal of *Healthy People 2010* as it
   relates to IPV (the number they want to see
   IPV decreased to)

   a. 4 per 1000 women per year

   b. 3

   c. 25%

   d. 45%

   e. 5%

   f. 4.8 million per year

   g. 30%

Historically, women have often been treated inhumanely. This continues even today. Based on information from the textbook, please select true or false for each of the following questions.

2. In ancient Roman times, women were provided fair and equal treatment in relation to acts of adultery and public drunkenness.
   a. True
   b. False ⟵ circled

3. As late as 2002, women in some Middle-Eastern cultures could legally be stoned to death or raped as punishment.
   a. True ⟵ circled
   b. False

4. Until 1870, abuse of one's wife was legal in the United States.
   a. True ⟵ circled
   b. False

5. Mental illness can be blamed for the majority of violent acts against women.
   a. True
   b. False

6. Children who are abused are more like to abuse as adults compared with children who have never been abused.
   a. True
   b. False

7. Violent episodes are greater among _____ and those with low-prestige jobs.

   _____ and _____ women report the highest rates of IPV in the United States.

Exercise 2

 CD-ROM Activity

 45 minutes

- Sign in to work at Pacific View Regional Hospital on the Obstetrics Floor for Period of Care 1. (*Note*: If you are already in the virtual hospital from a previous exercise, click on **Leave the Floor** and then **Restart the Program** to get to the sign-in window.)
- From the Patient List, select Dorothy Grant.
- Click on Go to **Nurses' Station**.
- Click on **Chart**.
- Click on the chart for Room **201**.
- Click on the **Nursing Admission** tab.

 In addition to reading about Dorothy Grant's perspective on the abusive relationship she has experienced, review the characteristics of battered women found on pages 135-136 in the textbook.

1. What is the reality of Dorothy Grant's situation? How does that correlate with the textbook reading?

→ • Still in Dorothy Grant's chart, review the **History and Physical** and the **Nursing Admission** as needed to answer question 2.

2. According to the textbook, battered women have certain characteristics. For each characteristic listed below and on the next page, discuss how Dorothy Grant compares with the textbook descriptions. Base your answers on what you have learned about the patient so far in your chart review. (*Note:* You will return to this list to add follow-up findings after viewing the 0810 video interaction between Dorothy Grant and the nurse.)

Financially dependent

Few resources/support systems

Blame themselves for what has taken place

State that they are not "good enough"

Bonding occurs out of fear and helplessness

Low self-esteem

History of domestic violence in their family

Fear societal rejection

Strong nurturing, yielding personality

Tolerate control from others easily

Attempt to avoid arousing anger in the abuser

Experience deliberate/repeated physical or sexual assault

- Click on **Return to Nurses' Station**.
- Click on Room **201** at the bottom of the screen.
- Click on the **Patient Care**.
- Click on **Nurse-Client Interactions**. (*Note:* Make notes as you watch the following video.)
- Select and view the video titled **0810: Monitoring/Patient Support**. (*Note*: If this video is not available, check the virtual clock to see whether enough time has elapsed. The video cannot be viewed before its specified time.)

3. In the video interaction what does Dorothy Grant verbalize that she should do to help prevent the violence?

4. In the video, what are the patient's concerns at the moment?

5. Return to question 2 and review your answers, keeping in mind what you have learned through the 0810 nurse-client interaction. Would you change any of your answers based on this observation? If so, what would you add or change?

Exercise 3

 CD-ROM Activity

 10 minutes

- Sign in to work at Pacific View Regional Hospital on the Obstetrics Floor for Period of Care 3. (*Note*: If you are already in the virtual hospital from a previous exercise, click on **Leave the Floor** and then **Restart the Program** to get to the sign-in window.)
- From the Patient List, select Dorothy Grant.
- Click on **Go to Nurses' Station**.
- Click on **Chart**.
- Click on the chart for Room **201**.
- Click on **Consultations** and review the Psychiatric Consult and the Social Work Consult.

 Review the information regarding the myths and facts about intimate partner violence on page 137 in the textbook. Based on that information and your review of Dorothy Grant's chart, answer the following:

1. Dorothy Grant stays in the relationship because of _____ and _____.

2. The percentage of women who are battered during pregnancy is _____.

3. Based on the information provided, in what phase of the abuse cycle is Dorothy Grant?

4. According to the consults, Dorothy Grant has several options. What are some of the options that the social worker and psychiatric heath care provider can offer her or assist her with?

5. Battering escalates or begins during pregnancy.
   a. True
   b. False

6. Dorothy Grant's husband blames her for the pregnancy.
   a. True
   b. False

7. Dorothy Grant stays in the relationship because likes to be beaten and deliberately provokes the attacks on occasion.
   a. True
   b. False

Exercise 4

 CD-ROM Activity

 10 minutes

- Sign in to work at Pacific View Regional Hospital on the Obstetrics Floor for Period of Care 4. (*Note*: If you are already in the virtual hospital from a previous exercise, click on **Leave the Floor** and then **Restart the Program** to get to the sign-in window.)
- From the Nurses' Station, click on **Kardex** and then on tab **201** to review Dorothy Grant's record.

1. What action was initiated on Wednesday to protect Dorothy Grant from her husband?

2. What care plan diagnoses are appropriate for this patient's current life situation?

3. What other disciplines have been contacted or consulted that will ensure continuity of care for Dorothy Grant as it relates to her abuse?

In your textbook, review pages 140-145 to assist in answering the following questions.

4. As a nurse caring for Dorothy Grant, what is your responsibility for reporting IPV?

5. What are the reporting requirements of the state in which you practice?

6. What are the resources available in your area for women who have experienced intimate partner violence?

Reproductive System Concerns, Contraception, and Infertility

 Reading Assignment: Reproductive Concerns (Chapter 7)
Contraception and Abortion (Chapter 9)
Infertility (Chapter 10)

Patients: Stacey Crider, Room 202
Kelly Brady, Room 203
Maggie Gardner, Room 204
Gabriela Valenzuela, Room 205
Laura Wilson, Room 206

Goal: Demonstrate an understanding of reproductive system concerns, contraception options and infertility.

Objectives:

- Identify reproductive concerns that can occur.
- Differentiate among the varying types of contraception available.
- Identify various methods of testing and treatment options that can be used for couples experiencing infertility concerns.

Exercise 1

 CD-ROM Activity

 10 minutes

Review information on pages 155-156 in your textbook.

1. What is a normal length for a menstrual cycle?

2. What are the criteria required to diagnose an individual with amenorrhea?

➡ • Sign in to work at Pacific View Regional Hospital on the Obstetrics Floor for Period of Care 1. (*Note*: If you are already in the virtual hospital from a previous exercise, click on **Leave the Floor** and then **Restart the Program** to get to the sign-in window.)

• From the Patient List, select Stacey Crider.

• Click on **Go to Nurses' Station**.

• Click on **Chart** and then on **202**.

• Click on **History and Physical**.

• Review the patient's gynecologic history. (*Hint:* See the bottom of page 1.)

3. Does Stacey Crider meet the textbook criteria for amenorrhea?

4. What is her history?

5. List three things that can cause amenorrhea.

Exercise 2

 CD-ROM Activity

 20 minutes

 Review pages 220-236 in the textbook.

1. What is contraception?

2. Providing contraception doesn't necessarily mean preventing _____.

➡ • Sign in to work at Pacific View Regional Hospital on the Obstetrics Floor for Period of Care 1. (*Note*: If you are already in the virtual hospital from a previous exercise, click on **Leave the Floor** and then **Restart the Program** to get to the sign-in window.)

• From the Patient List, select Kelly Brady, Gabriela Valezuela, and Laura Wilson.

• Click on **Go to Nurses' Station**.

• Click on **Chart** and then on **203** for Kelly Brady's chart.

• Review the **History and Physical**.

• Repeat the previous two steps for Gabriela Valenzuela and Laura Wilson.

3. Based on your review of their charts, list the birth control method each of these women were using prior to their current pregnancy

Kelly Brady

Gabriela Valenzuela

Laura Wilson

Answer questions 4, 5, and 6 after reviewing the Legal Tip on page 221 of your textbook.

4. When assisting individuals with contraception, what needs to be reviewed by the nurse?

5. Gabriela Valenzuela is Catholic. Which method would be appropriate for the nurse to discuss with her?

6. What does this method rely on?

Review pages 232-236 in your textbook; then answer questions 7 and 8.

7. Kelly Brady desires to use oral contraceptives while breastfeeding to prevent pregnancy. Which type of oral contraception is appropriate for her to use? Why?

8. Laura Wilson is HIV-positive. What is the most appropriate form of birth control for her? Why?

Exercise 3

  CD-ROM Activity

20 minutes

 Review Chapter 10 in your textbook.

1. _____ of the reproductive age population has a problem with infertility.

2. At the age of _____ the incidence of infertility in women increases.

Maggie Gardner is 41 years old. Let's consider some of the options she had while attempting to get pregnant.

3. List four factors that affect female fertility.

4. List five factors that affect male fertility.

→ • Sign in to work at Pacific View Regional Hospital on the Obstetrics Floor for Period of Care 1. (*Note*: If you are already in the virtual hospital from a previous exercise, click on **Leave the Floor** and then **Restart the Program** to get to the sign-in window.)
   • From the Patient List, select Maggie Gardner.
   • Click on **Go to Nurses' Station**.
   • Click on **Chart** and then on **204**.
   • Review the **History and Physical**.

5. Maggie Gardner was married _____ years prior to conceiving the first time.

6. Based on the textbook reading, which of the following would Maggie Gardner have been diagnosed with if she had chosen to get treatment after a year of attempting to get pregnant?

   a. Primary infertility
   b. Secondary infertility

Review pages 250-255 in your textbook to answer the following questions.

7. What four tests can be completed on a female patient to determine the causes of infertility?

8. What two tests can be completed on a male patient to determine the causes of infertility?

9. What test is used to assess a couple to determine adequacy of coital technique?

10. What methods are available to assist an infertile couple in conceiving?

11. What methods did Maggie Gardner and her husband use to assist in getting pregnant? (*Hint*: Review the OB history in the History and Physical.)

Sexually Transmitted and Other Infections

 Reading Assignment: Sexually Transmitted and Other Infections (Chapter 8)

Patients: Stacey Crider, Room 202
Gabriela Valenzuela, Room 205
Laura Wilson, Room 206

Goal: Demonstrate understanding of the identification and management of selected sexually transmitted and other infections in pregnant women.

Objectives:

- Assess and plan care for a pregnant woman with bacterial vaginosis.
- Explain the importance of prophylactic Group B streptococcus treatment.
- Identify risk factors for acquiring HIV infection.
- Prioritize information to be included in patient teaching related to HIV infection.

In this lesson you will assess and evaluate the care provided to three hospitalized pregnant women, each of whom has a sexually transmitted infection (STI).

Exercise 1

 CD-ROM Activity

15 minutes

- Sign in to work at Pacific View Regional Hospital on the Obstetrics Floor for Period of Care 1. (*Note*: If you are already in the virtual hospital from a previous exercise, click on **Leave the Floor** and then **Restart the Program** to get to the sign-in window.)
- From the Patient List, select Stacey Crider.
- Click on **Go to Nurses' Station**.
- Click on **Chart** and then on chart for Room **202**.
- Click on **History and Physical**.

1. In the table below, describe Stacey Crider's vaginal discharge on admission. How does it compare with the description of bacterial vaginosis found on page 206 in the textbook?

	Stacey Crider's Discharge	Textbook Description
Appearance		
Amount		
Odor		

2. Consult Table 8-5 on page 207 in the textbook. How is bacterial vaginosis diagnosed?

3. Which medications are recommended for treating bacterial vaginosis during pregnancy?

→ • Now click on **Physician's Orders** in the chart.
   • Scroll down to the admitting physician's orders on Tuesday at 0630.

4. What are Stacey Crider's admission diagnoses?

5. Explain how Stacey Crider's admission diagnoses are likely to be related.

6. Which medication did Stacey Crider's physician order to treat her bacterial vaginosis?

7. Assume that Stacey Crider is discharged home on day 4 of the prescribed treatment with the medication you identified in question 6. What specific information about this medication should she be taught? (*Hint*: Check page 208 in the textbook.)

Exercise 2

 CD-ROM Activity

 15 minutes

- Sign in to work at Pacific View Regional Hospital on the Obstetrics Floor for Period of Care 1. (*Note*: If you are already in the virtual hospital from a previous exercise, click on **Leave the Floor** and then **Restart the Program** to get to the sign-in window.)
- From the Patient List, select Gabriela Valenzuela.
- Click on **Go to Nurses' Station**.
- Click on **Chart** and then on chart for Room **205**.
- Click on **History and Physical** and scroll to the plan at the end of this document.

1. What is the medical plan of care for Gabriela Valenzuela?

2. Is Gabriela Valenzuela known to be positive for Group B streptococcus (GBS)?

 Read about Group B streptococcus on page 209 in your textbook; then answer questions 3 through 6.

3. List risk factors for neonatal GBS infection. Which risk factor applies to Gabriela Valenzuela?

4. Since pregnant women with GBS in the vagina are almost always asymptomatic, why does Gabriela Valenzuela need to be treated for this organism?

 • Click on **Physician's Orders**.
- Scroll to the admission orders written Tuesday at 2100.

5. What medication/dosage/frequency will Gabriela Valenzuela receive for Group B strep prophylaxis?

6. How does this order compare with the treatment regimen recommended in your textbook?

Exercise 3

 CD-ROM Activity

 35 minutes

- Sign in to work at Pacific View Regional Hospital on the Obstetrics Floor for Period of Care 1. (*Note*: If you are already in the virtual hospital from a previous exercise, click on **Leave the Floor** and then **Restart the Program** to get to the sign-in window.)
- From the Patient List, select Laura Wilson.
- Click on **Go to Nurses' Station**.
- Click on **Chart** and then on chart for Room **206**.
- Click on **Nursing Admission**.

1. What risk factors for acquiring an STI are identified on Laura Wilson's Nursing Admission form?

 2. List specific risk factors for acquiring HIV infection. (*Hint:* See page 203 in the textbook.) Underline the risk factors that are present in Laura Wilson's history.

3. What did the admitting nurse document about Laura Wilson's knowledge and acceptance of her HIV diagnosis?

 • Click on **Return to Nurses' Station**.
 • Click on **Patient Care**.
 • Click on **Nurse-Client Interactions**.
 • Select and view the video titled **0800: Teaching—HIV in Pregnancy**. (*Note*: If this video is not available, check the virtual clock to see whether enough time has elapsed. The video cannot be viewed before its specified time.)

4. Does Laura Wilson appear to be fully aware of the implications of HIV infection? State the rationale for your answer.

5. What coping mechanism is Laura Wilson exhibiting in the video interaction?

 • Click on **Chart**.
 • Click on **Nursing Admission**

6. Laura Wilson needs education on all of the following topics. Which would you choose to teach her about at this time?

_____ Safer sex

_____ Medication side effects and importance of compliance

_____ Need for medical follow-up and medication for the baby

_____ Impact of HIV on birth plans

7. Give a rationale for your answer to question 6.

LESSON 6

Assessment of Risk Factors in Pregnancy, Including Maternal and Fetal Nutrition

 Reading Assignment: Maternal and Fetal Nutrition (Chapter 15)
Assessment of Risk Factors (Chapter 29)

Patients: Kelly Brady, Room 203
Maggie Gardner, Room 204
Laura Wilson, Room 206

Goal: Demonstrate an understanding of assessment of risk factors in pregnancy, including maternal and fetal nutritional aspects.

Objectives:

- Identify appropriate interventions for maintaining appropriate maternal and fetal nutrition.
- Differentiate among the varying types of assessment techniques that can be used with pregnant patients—both low- and high-risk patients.
- Identify various methods of testing that can be used in high-risk pregnancies.

Exercise 1

 CD-ROM Activity

15 minutes

- Sign in to work at Pacific View Regional Hospital on the Obstetrics Floor for Period of Care 1. (*Note*: If you are already in the virtual hospital from a previous exercise, click on **Leave the Floor** and then **Restart the Program** to get to the sign-in window.)
- From the Patient List, select Maggie Gardner
- Click on **Go to Nurses' Station**.
- Click on **Chart** and then on **204**.
- Click on the **Laboratory Reports**.

Review pages 918-920 in the textbook for information regarding anemia.

1. What were Maggie Gardner's hemoglobin and hematocrit levels on admission?

→ • Click on **History and Physical**.

2. What puts Maggie Gardner at a greater risk for developing anemia than the average pregnancy patient? (*Hint*: Review the Genetic Screening section of her History and Physical.)

3. What percentage of women are affected by anemia during their pregnancy?

4. What complication do women with anemia experience at a higher rate than those without anemia?

5. What is a normal hematocrit level for women who are pregnant?

6. What assessments need to be performed by the nurse at each visit specifically related to an anemia diagnosis?

7. According to Table 15-1 in the textbook, what are some good sources of iron that you could instruct Maggie Gardner to add to her diet?

8. Maggie Gardner is not on iron supplementation at this time; however, list three things that you could teach her about iron supplementation. (*Hint*: See the Teaching for Self-Care box on page 379 of your textbook.)

Exercise 2

CD-ROM Activity

15 minutes

Review pages 811-816 in the textbook.

1. A high-risk pregnancy is one in which the life or health of _____ or

   _____ is jeopardized by a _____ coincidental with or unique to pregnancy.

- Sign in to work at Pacific View Regional Hospital on the Obstetrics Floor for Period of Care 3. (*Note*: If you are already in the virtual hospital from a previous exercise, click on **Leave the Floor** and then **Restart the Program** to get to the sign-in window.)
- From the Patient List, select Kelly Brady, Maggie Gardner, and Laura Wilson.
- Click on **Go to Nurses' Station**.
- Click on **Chart**.
- For each of these three patients, open the chart and review the **History and Physical** as needed to answer question 2.

2. After reviewing the History and Physical, list the things that place each of these patients at risk during their pregnancy.

Kelly Brady

Maggie Gardner

Laura Wilson

Before answering questions 3 through 7, review Box 29-3 in your textbook for information regarding specific categories of high-risk factors.

3. A patient who consumes large amounts of caffeine may have a slight decrease in

_____ in her newborn.

4. The exact effects of alcohol in pregnancy are not known. However, it can result in

_____, _____, and _____.

5. Young mothers (under 15 years old) have a _____ higher mortality rate than those older than 20 years.

6. _____ and _____ have a higher incidence with the first birth.

7. African-American babies have the highest rates of _____ and

_____. The infant mortality among African Americans is more than

_____ that of Caucasians.

Exercise 3

 CD-ROM Activity

 10 minutes

 Review information regarding ultrasounds on pages 818-822 in the textbook.

1. List three things that ultrasounds are used for.

2. What are two forms of ultrasound? When are they used?

 • Sign in to work at Pacific View Regional Hospital on the Obstetrics Floor for Period of Care 3. (*Note*: If you are already in the virtual hospital from a previous exercise, click on **Leave the Floor** and then **Restart the Program** to get to the sign-in window.)
• From the Patient List, select Maggie Gardner
• Click on **Go to Nurses' Station**.
• Click on **Chart** and then on **204**.
• Click on **Diagnostic Reports**.

3. What type of ultrasound is Maggie Gardner having?

4. Based on the ultrasound findings, how large is her baby?

5. List three abnormalities found on the ultrasound in regard to the placenta.

6. What is the impression from Maggie Gardner's ultrasound in terms of the fetus and the placenta?

7. What are the recommendations regarding follow-up?

Exercise 4

 CD-ROM Activity

 15 minutes

 Biophysical profile is another very important assessment tool used with patients who are experiencing a high-risk pregnancy. Review information regarding biophysical profiles on pages 822-823 in the textbook.

1. What are the five items that are assessed on a biophysical profile?

2. Abnormalities in the amniotic fluid index are frequently associated with _____.

3. The biophysical profile is an accurate indicator of impending _____.

4. The normal score on a biophysical profile is _____.

→ • Sign in to work at Pacific View Regional Hospital on the Obstetrics Floor for Period of Care 3. (*Note*: If you are already in the virtual hospital from a previous exercise, click on **Leave the Floor** and then **Restart the Program** to get to the sign-in window.)

• From the Patient List, select Kelly Brady.

• Click on **Go to Nurses' Station**.

• Click on **Chart** and then on **203**.

• Click on **Diagnostic Reports**.

5. What is the estimated gestational age of Kelly Brady's fetus?

6. What is the amniotic fluid index as indicated on the report?

7. How does this correlate with the normal index as listed in the textbook?

8. What is the score on the biophysical profile?

9. Based on the information you have learned through your review of the textbook, what does this score indicate?

Nursing Care During Pregnancy

/OD **Reading Assignment:** Nursing Care During Pregnancy (Chapter 16)

Patients: Kelly Brady, Room 203
                  Maggie Gardner, Room 204
                  Laura Wilson, Room 206

Goal: Demonstrate an understanding of the nursing care provided to women during normal pregnancy.

Objectives:

- Identify common physical and psychologic findings associated with each trimester of pregnancy.
- Describe differences in the normal pregnancy changes experienced by adolescent and older mothers.

In this lesson you will identify physical and psychologic pregnancy changes as they occur in three women at different gestational ages.

Exercise 1

 CD-ROM Activity

 20 minutes

 Read the section on Diagnosis of Pregnancy on pages 397-398 in your textbook.

1. List the subjective presumptive indicators of pregnancy identified in your textbook.

→ • Sign in to work at Pacific View Regional Hospital on the Obstetrics Floor for Period of Care 1. (*Note*: If you are already in the virtual hospital from a previous exercise, click on **Leave the Floor** and then **Restart the Program** to get to the sign-in window.)
• From the Patient List, select Maggie Gardner, Room 204.
• Click on **Go to Nurses' Station**.
• Click on **Charts** and then on the chart for Room **204**.
• Click on **Nursing Admission**.

2. Place an X beside each of the subjective presumptive indicators of pregnancy that applies to Maggie Gardner, according to the Nursing Admission.

_____ Amenorrhea

_____ Nausea/vomiting

_____ Breast tenderness

_____ Urinary frequency

_____ Fatigue

_____ Quickening

3. Uterine enlargement is considered a _____ indicator of pregnancy.

4. List three positive indicators of pregnancy.

→ • Click on **Return to Nurses' Station**.
• Click on Room **204** at the bottom of the screen.
• Click on **Patient Care**.
• Perform a focused physical assessment by clicking on **Abdomen** and then on **Reproductive**.

5. What probable and positive pregnancy indicators are found in the abdominal assessment?

Probable

Positive

Read the section on Estimating Date of Birth on page 398 in your textbook.

→ • Click on **Chart** and then on **204**.
  • Click on **Nursing Admission**.
  • Scroll to the Pregnancy section on page 5.

6. What is recorded as Maggie Gardner's LMP?

7. Using Nagele's Rule, calculate Maggie Gardner's EDB. Explain how you calculated this date.

Exercise 2

CD-ROM Activity

20 minutes

Laura Wilson and Kelly Brady represent age extremes among women of childbearing age. Read the section on Adolescent Pregnancy on pages 441-442 in your textbook.

1. About 1 million adolescents in the United States, or _____ of every _____ girls, become

   pregnant each year. Nearly _____ of these pregnancies end in abortion. _____

   currently have the highest birth rate. Of girls who become pregnant, 1 in 6 will have a

   repeat pregnancy within _____.

2. List common characteristics of pregnant adolescents, according to your textbook.

 • Sign in to work at Pacific View Regional Hospital on the Obstetrics Floor for Period of Care 4. (*Note*: If you are already in the virtual hospital from a previous exercise, click on **Leave the Floor** and then **Restart the Program** to get to the sign-in window.)
 • Click on **Charts** and then on **206** for Laura Wilson's chart.
 • Click on **Nursing Admission**.

3. Based on your chart review, how does Laura Wilson compare with the textbook profile of the pregnant adolescent? Explain how each of the characteristics you listed in question 2 applies (or does not apply) to Laura Wilson.

Read the section on Older Primiparous Women on page 443 in your textbook.

4. List common characteristics of older primiparous women, according to your textbook.

 • Click on **Return to Nurses' Station**.
 • Click on **Chart** and then on **203** for Kelly Brady's chart.
 • Click on **Nursing Admission**.

5. Based on your chart review, how does Kelly Brady compare with the textbook profile of the older primiparous woman? Explain how each of the characteristics you listed in question 4 applies (or does not apply) to Kelly Brady.

6. Women 35 years and older are more likely than younger primiparas to have

_____ infants, _____, and _____.

Exercise 3

CD-ROM Activity

15 minutes

- Sign in to work at Pacific View Regional Hospital on the Obstetrics Floor for Period of Care 4. (*Note*: If you are already in the virtual hospital from a previous exercise, click on **Leave the Floor** and then **Restart the Program** to get to the sign-in window.)
- Click on **Return to Nurses' Station**.
- Click on **Chart** and then on the chart for Room **204** for Maggie Gardner's chart.
- Click on **Nursing Admission**.

1. What is Maggie Gardner's gestational age?

2. Maggie Gardner is in the _____ trimester of pregnancy.

→ • Click on **Chart** and then on **206** for Laura Wilson's chart.
- Click on **Nursing Admission**.

3. What is Laura Wilson's gestational age?

4. Laura Wilson is in the _____ trimester of pregnancy.

Read the section on Adaptation to Pregnancy on pages 398-406 in your textbook.

5. Match each of the following behaviors in the pregnant woman with the trimester of pregnancy in which it is most likely to occur.

_____ Has fantasies about the fetus

_____ Is more interested in relationships with her mother and other women who are or have been pregnant

_____ Demonstrates emotional lability

_____ Ready for the pregnancy to end

_____ Has ambivalent feelings

_____ May experience increased desire for sex because of increased pelvic congestion

_____ Realistically prepares for birth and parenting the child

a. Second trimester

b. Third trimester

c. Throughout pregnancy

LESSON 8

Nursing Care During Labor and Birth

Reading Assignment: Nursing Care During Labor (Chapter 21)

Patients: Dorothy Grant, Room 201
Gabriela Valenzuela, Room 205
Laura Wilson, Room 206

Goal: Demonstrate an understanding of the normal labor and birth process.

Objectives:

- Assess and identify signs and symptoms present in each phase of Stage I labor.
- Describe appropriate nursing care for the patient in Stage I labor.

In this lesson you will plan and evaluate care for three patients in Stage I labor.

Exercise 1

 CD-ROM Activity

 20 minutes

- Sign in to work at Pacific View Regional Hospital on the Obstetrics Floor for Period of Care 1. (*Note*: If you are already in the virtual hospital from a previous exercise, click on **Leave the Floor** and then **Restart the Program** to get to the sign-in window.)
- From the Patient List, select Dorothy Grant, Room 201
- Click on **Go to Nurses' Station**.
- Click on **Charts** and then on the chart for Room **201**.
- Click on **Nurse's Notes**.
- Scroll to the entry for 0730.

1. List the findings from Dorothy Grant's most recent cervical exam.

➡ • Click on **Return to Nurses' Station**.
- Click on **EPR**.
- Click **Login**.
- Select **201** as the patient's room and **Obstetrics** as the category.

2. At 0700, what was the recorded frequency and duration of Dorothy Grant's contractions?

➡ • Now select **Vital Signs** as the category.

3. At 0700, what was Dorothy Grant's recorded pain level?

 Consult Table 21-1 on page 549 in your textbook.

4. At this time, which phase of Stage I labor is Dorothy Grant in?

5. For each specific assessment listed below, compare the typical findings for latent labor with Dorothy Grant's current condition.

Assessment	Typical Findings for Latent Labor	Findings for Dorothy Grant
Cervical dilation		
Contraction frequency		
Contraction duration		
Contraction intensity		

 Consult Table 21-3 on page 554 in your textbook.

6. List the typical behaviors in latent phase labor.

- Click on **Exit EPR**.
- Click on **201** at the bottom of the screen.
- Click on **Patient Care**.
- Click on **Nurse-Client Interactions**.
- Select and view the video titled **0810: Monitoring/Patient Support**. (*Note*: If this video is not available, check the virtual clock to see whether enough time has elapsed. The video cannot be viewed before its specified time.)

7. Based on the video interaction, place an X next to each characteristic that is true of Dorothy Grant.

_____ Excited

_____ Thoughts center on self, labor, and baby

_____ Some apprehension

_____ Pain fairly well controlled

_____ Alert

_____ Follows directions readily

_____ Open to instructions

Exercise 2

 CD-ROM Activity

 45 minutes

- Sign in to work at Pacific View Regional Hospital on the Obstetrics Floor for Period of Care 2. (*Note*: If you are already in the virtual hospital from a previous exercise, click on **Leave the Floor** and then **Restart the Program** to get to the sign-in window.)
- From the Patient List, select Gabriela Valenzuela.

 Read the sections on Physical Nursing Care During Labor and Supportive Care During Labor and Birth, pages 569-580 in your textbook.

- Click on **Go to Nurses' Station**.
- Click on **Chart** and then on the chart for Room **205**.
- Click on **Nurse's Notes**.
- Scroll back to the entry for 0800.

1. What was Gabriela Valenzuela's condition at this time? What phase of labor was she experiencing?

Consult Table 21-1 on page 549 in your textbook.

2. As Gabriela Valenzuela progresses in labor, which phase will she enter next?

3. List the common interventions for active phase labor.

→ • Still in the Nurse's Notes, scroll to the entry for 1140.

4. How is Gabriela Valenzuela tolerating labor at this time? Do you believe she has entered active phase?

5. How could you determine for certain which phase of labor Gabriela Valenzuela is currently experiencing?

→ • Click on **Return to Nurses' Station**.
• Click on **205** at the bottom of the screen.
• Click on **Patient Care**.
• Click on **Nurse-Client Interactions**.
• Select and view the video titled: **1140: Intervention—Bleeding, Comfort**. (*Note*: If this video is not available, check the virtual clock to see whether enough time has elapsed. The video cannot be viewed before its specified time.)

6. Based on the video interaction, place an X next to each intervention suggested or implemented by the nurse.

_____ Limit assessment techniques to between contractions

_____ Assist patient to cope with contractions

_____ Encourage patient to help her maintain breathing techniques

_____ Use comfort measures

_____ Encourage voluntary muscle relaxation and use of effleurage

_____ Apply counterpressure to sacrococcygeal area

_____ Offer encouragement and praise

_____ Keep patient aware of progress

_____ Offer analgesics as ordered

_____ Check bladder; encourage voiding

_____ Give oral care; offer fluids, food, ice chips as ordered

→ • Click on **Patient Care**.
 • Click on **Nurse-Client Interactions**.
 • Select and view the video titled: **1155: Evaluation—Comfort Measures**. (*Note*: If this video is not available, check the virtual clock to see whether enough time has elapsed. The video cannot be viewed before its specified time.)

7. Based on the video interaction, place an X next to each intervention suggested or implemented by the nurse and/or Gabriela Valenzuela's husband.

_____ Limit assessment techniques to between contractions

_____ Assist patient to cope with contractions

_____ Encourage patient to help her maintain breathing techniques

_____ Use comfort measures

_____ Assist with position changes

_____ Encourage voluntary muscle relaxation and use of effleurage

_____ Apply counterpressure to sacrococcygeal area

_____ Offer encouragement and praise

_____ Keep patient aware of progress

_____ Offer analgesics as ordered

_____ Check bladder; encourage voiding

_____ Give oral care; offer fluids, food, ice chips as ordered

Exercise 3

  CD-ROM Activity

 30 minutes

Let's jump ahead to Period of Care 4. Remember, you are not able to visit patients during this shift, but you have access to all patient records. First, we'll review Dorothy Grant's status.

- Sign in to work at Pacific View Regional Hospital on the Obstetrics Floor for Period of Care 4. (*Note*: If you are already in the virtual hospital from a previous exercise, click on **Leave the Floor** and then **Restart the Program** to get to the sign-in window.)
- From the Nurses' Station, click on **EPR** and then on **Login**.
- In the Patient drop-down menu, select **201** for Dorothy Grant's records. Choose **Obstetrics** as the category.
- Scroll to review the entries for Wednesday 1800 and 1815.

1. What are the findings from Dorothy Grant's cervical exam at 1815?

 Consult Table 21-1 on page 549 in your textbook.

2. At this time, which phase of Stage I labor is Dorothy Grant experiencing?

3. Complete the table below, listing typical findings for each assessment in the transition phase of Stage I labor.

Assessment	Typical Findings
Cervical dilation	
Contraction frequency	
Contraction duration	
Contraction intensity	

Consult Table 21-3 on page 554 in your textbook.

4. List the typical behaviors seen in patients experiencing the transition phase of labor.

- Click on **Exit EPR**.
- Click on **Chart** and then on **201** for Dorothy Grant's chart.
- Click on **Nurse's Notes**.
- Read the notes recorded at 1800, 1815, and 1830 on Wednesday.

5. Based on information recorded in the EPR and Nurse's Notes, place an X next to each behavior Dorothy Grant exhibited during transition phase of labor.

_____ Severe pain

_____ Frustration; fear of loss of control

_____ Writhing with contractions

_____ Nausea/vomiting

_____ Perspiration

_____ Shaking or tremors

_____ Feeling the need to defecate

Now let's review Laura Wilson's status.

- Click on **Return to Nurses' Station**.
- Click on **EPR** and then on **Login**.
- Select **206** as the patient's room number and **Vital Signs** as the category.

1. Below, record Laura Wilson's assessment findings from 1815 on Wednesday.

Pain location

Pain intensity

- Now select **Obstetrics** as the category.

2. Below, record Laura Wilson's 1830 assessment findings.

Contraction frequency

Contraction duration

- Scroll back through earlier Obstetrics entries until you locate the results of Laura Wilson's most recent cervical exam.

3. When was Laura Wilson's most recent cervical examination performed? What were the results?

• Click on **Exit EPR**.
- Click on **Chart** and then on **206** for Laura Wilson's chart.
- Click **Nurse's Notes**.
- Scroll to the note for Wednesday 1830.

4. According to this note, what event occurred at 1815?

 Read the Assessment of Amniotic Membranes and Fluid section on pages 565-567 in your textbook. Also read the Procedure Box on Tests for Rupture of Membranes on page 547.

5. List the immediate nursing actions appropriate for the situation you identified in question 4.

6. According to the Nurse's Notes and your textbook recommendations, did Laura Wilson's nurse handle this situation appropriately? Explain.

7. Based only on the information you have learned about Laura Wilson during this exercise, write the nursing diagnosis that you consider to be of highest priority for her at this time.

8. List several nursing interventions for the nursing diagnosis you wrote in question 7.

Management of Discomfort

👓 **Reading Assignment:** Management of Discomfort (Chapter 19)

Patients: Kelly Brady, Room 203
Gabriela Valenzuela, Room 205
Laura Wilson, Room 206

Goal: Demonstrate an understanding of the normal labor and birth process.

Objectives:

* Assess and identify factors that influence pain perception.
* Describe selected nonpharmacologic and pharmacologic measures for pain management during labor and birth.

In this lesson you will compare and contrast the pain management strategies used with three patients during labor and birth.

Exercise 1

 CD-ROM Activity

 45 minutes

* Sign in to work at Pacific View Regional Hospital on the Obstetrics Floor for Period of Care 1. (*Note*: If you are already in the virtual hospital from a previous exercise, click on **Leave the Floor** and then **Restart the Program** to get to the sign-in window.)
* From the Patient List, select Laura Wilson.
* Click on **Get Report**.

1. What is Laura Wilson's condition when you assume care for her, according to the change-of-shift report?

• Click on **Go to Nurses' Station**.
  • Click on Room **206** at the bottom of the screen.
  • Read the **Initial Observations**.

2. What is your impression of Laura Wilson's condition?

 • Click on **Patient Care**.
  • Click on **Nurse-Client Interactions**.
  • Select and view the video titled **0730: Patient Assessment**. (*Note*: If this video is not available, check the virtual clock to see whether enough time has elapsed. The video cannot be viewed before its specified time.)

3. What is Laura Wilson's assessment of her current condition? How does this compare with the information you received from the shift report and the Initial Observations summary?

• Click on **Chart** and then on **206**.
  • Click on **Nursing Admission**.

4. List Laura Wilson's admission diagnoses. (*Hint:* See page 1 of the Nursing Admission form.)

5. What is your perception of Laura Wilson's behavior? What data did you collect during this exercise that led you to this perception?

6. Think about the following questions and then discuss your ideas with your classmates: Do your personal values and beliefs contribute to your perception of Laura Wilson's behavior? If so, how? What nursing interventions might help to overcome your personal biases when dealing with Laura Wilson?

 Read the section on Factors Influencing Pain Response on pages 489-491 in your textbook.

 Continue reviewing Laura Wilson's **Nursing Admission** form as needed to answer question 7.

7. Each woman's pain during childbirth is unique and is influenced by a variety of factors. For each factor listed below, explain how that factor influences pain perception (in the middle column). Then, in the right column, list data from Laura Wilson's Nursing Admission that support how that factor might relate to her particular pain perception.

Factor	Typical Effect on Pain Perception	Laura Wilson's Supporting Data
Anxiety		
Previous experience		
Childbirth preparation		
Support		

Exercise 2

 CD-ROM Activity

 45 minutes

- Sign in to work at Pacific View Regional Hospital on the Obstetrics Floor for Period of Care 2. (*Note*: If you are already in the virtual hospital from a previous exercise, click on **Leave the Floor** and then **Restart the Program** to get to the sign-in window.)
- From the Patient List, select Gabriela Valenzuela.

 Read the sections on Relaxing and Breathing Techniques (pages 492-494), Touch and Massage (page 497), and Systemic Analgesia (pages 498-501) in your textbook.

1. Focusing and relaxation techniques allow a woman in labor to rest and conserve energy by

   _____. While focusing on an object during a contraction, the

   woman _____ to reduce her _____.

   Varying breathing techniques are used to provide _____. All patterns begin and

   end with a _____.

2. Touch can communicate _____, _____, and _____.

   When using touch, it is important to determine the _____.

   Hand, back, and foot massage may be very effective in _____

   and _____.

 • Click on **Get Report**.

3. Is Gabriela Valenzuela in labor at this time? Give a rationale for your answer.

 • Click on **Return to Patient List**.
- Click **Go to Nurses' Station**.
- Click on Room **205** at the bottom of the screen.
- Click on **Patient Care**.
- Click on **Nurse-Client Interactions**.
- Select and view the video titled **1140: Intervention—Bleeding, Comfort**. (*Note*: If this video is not available, check the virtual clock to see whether enough time has elapsed. The video cannot be viewed before its specified time.)
- Click on **Chart**.
- Click on **Nurse's Notes**.
- Scroll to the entry for 1140 on Wednesday.

4. How is Gabriela Valenzuela tolerating labor at this time?

5. What pain interventions does the nurse implement at this time?

Read the Medication Guide on fentanyl on page 500 in your textbook.

6. What is the action of this drug?

Let's begin the process for preparing and administering Gabriela Valenzuela's fentanyl dose.

→ • First, click on **Medication Room**.
  • Next, click on **MAR** and then on tab **205**.
  • Scroll down to the PRN Medication Administration Record for Wednesday.

7. What is the ordered dose of fentanyl?

→ • Click on **Return to Medication Room**.
  • Click on **Automated System**.
  • Click on **Login**.
  • In box 1, click on **Gabriela Valenzuela, 205**.
  • In box 2, click on **Automated System Drawer A-F**.
  • Click on **Fentanyl citrate**.
  • Click on **Put Medication on Tray**.
  • Click on **Close Drawer**.
  • Click on **View Medication Room**.
  • Click on **Preparation**.
  • Click on **Prepare** and follow the Preparation Wizard prompts to complete preparation of Gabriela Valenzuela's Fentanyl dose. When the Wizard stops requesting information, click **Finish**.
  • Click on **Return to Medication Room**.
  • Click on **205** to go to the patient's room.

8. What additional assessments must be completed before you give Gabriela Valenzuela's medication?

9. Why is it important to check Gabriela Valenzuela's respirations prior to giving the dose of fentanyl?

10. What safety precautions should be in effect for Gabriela Valenzuela after she receives this dose of fentanyl?

→ • Click on **Patient Care** and then **Medication Administration**.
 • Click on **Review Your Medications** and verify the accuracy of your preparation. Click **Return to Room 205**.
 • Next, click the down arrow next to **Select** and choose **Administer**.
 • Follow the Administration Wizard prompts to administer Gabriela Valenzuela's fentanyl dose. (*Note:* Click **Yes** when asked whether to document this administration in the MAR.)
 • When the Wizard stops asking questions, click **Finish**.
 • Still in Gabriela Valenzuela's room, click on **Patient Care**.
 • Click on **Nurse-Client Interactions**.
 • Select and view the video titled: **1155: Evaluation—Comfort Measures**. (*Note*: If this video is not available, check the virtual clock to see whether enough time has elapsed. The video cannot be viewed before its specified time.)

11. How effective were the interventions you identified in question 5?

12. Gabriela Valenzuela is experiencing _____. _____

is responsible for the dizziness as well as other side effects, including

_____, _____, and

_____.

13. What interventions does the nurse suggest to deal with this problem? List other interventions described in your textbook.

 At the end of the 1155 video, Gabriela Valenzuela states that she "doesn't want any needles" in her back. Learn more about this by reading the section on Epidural Anesthesia/Analgesia on pages 505-506 in your textbook.

14. What could you tell Gabriela Valenzuela to help her make an informed decision about anesthesia for labor? Below, list advantages and disadvantages of epidural anesthesia.

Advantages   **Disadvantages**

Before leaving this period of care, let's see how you did preparing and administering the patient's medication.

 • Click on **Leave the Floor**.
  • Click on **Look at Your Preceptor's Evaluation**.
  • Click on **Medication Scorecard** and review the evaluation. How did you do? (*Hint:* For a quick refresher on reading your Medication Scorecard, see page 22 in the **Getting Started** section of this workbook. For a more detailed tour on preparing and administering medications and interpreting your Scorecard, see pages 26-31 and 36-40.)

Exercise 3

 CD-ROM Activity

 20 minutes

 Read the section on General Anesthesia on page 508 in your textbook.

- Sign in to work at Pacific View Regional Hospital on the Obstetrics Floor for Period of Care 4. (*Note*: If you are already in the virtual hospital from a previous exercise, click on **Leave the Floor** and then **Restart the Program** to get to the sign-in window.)
- From the Nurses' Station, click on **Chart** and then on **203** for Kelly Brady's chart.
- Click on **Nurse's Notes**.
- Scroll to the entry for 1730 on Wednesday.

 1. Why does the anesthesiologist plan to use general anesthesia during Kelly Brady's cesarean section? (*Hint*: Read the section on Contraindications to Subarachnoid and Epidural Block on page 507 in your textbook.)

2. Why is Kelly Brady upset about receiving general anesthesia for her surgery?

 • Click on **Physician's Orders**.
- Review the entry for Wednesday at 1540.

3. What preoperative medications are ordered for Kelly Brady?

 • Click on **Return to Nurses' Station**.
- Click on the **Drug** icon in the lower left corner of your screen to access the Drug Guide.
- Use the Search box or the scroll bar to read about each of the drugs you listed in question 3.

4. All of these medications are given preoperatively to help prevent aspiration pneumonia. Using information from the Drug Guide and from the section on General Anesthesia in your textbook, match each of the medications below with the description of how it specifically works to prevent aspiration pneumonia.

_____ Sodium citrate/citric acid (Bicitra)   a. Decreases the production of gastric acid.

_____ Metoclopramide (Reglan)   b. Prevents nausea and vomiting and accelerates gastric emptying

_____ Ranitidine (Zantac)

c. Neutralizes acidic stomach contents

5. During general anesthesia, a short-acting barbiturate is administered to

_____. A muscle relaxer is then given to

_____. A low concentration of a volatile halogenated agent

may be administered to _____.

6. How would you expect general anesthesia to affect Kelly Brady's baby? Why?

LESSON **10** ———————————————

Hypertensive Disorders in Pregnancy

 Reading Assignment: Hypertensive Disorders in Pregnancy (Chapter 30)

Patient: Kelly Brady, Room 203

Goal: Demonstrate an understanding of the identification and management of selected hypertensive complications of pregnancy.

Objectives:

- Assess and identify signs and symptoms present in the patient with severe preeclampsia.
- Explain how common signs and symptoms present in the patient with severe preeclampsia relate to the underlying pathophysiology of this disease.
- Identify the patient who has developed HELLP syndrome.
- Describe routine nursing care for the patient with severe preeclampsia who is receiving magnesium sulfate.

In this lesson you will assess and plan care for a patient with severe preeclampsia who then develops HELLP syndrome and delivers at 26 2/7 weeks gestation.

Exercise 1

 CD-ROM Activity

20 minutes

- Sign in to work at Pacific View Regional Hospital on the Obstetrics Floor for Period of Care 3. (*Note*: If you are already in the virtual hospital from a previous exercise, click on **Leave the Floor** and then **Restart the Program** to get to the sign-in window.)
- From the Patient List, select Kelly Brady.
- Click on **Go to Nurses' Station**.
- Click on **Charts** and then on the chart for Room **203**.
- Click on **History and Physical**.

1. What was Kelly Brady's admission diagnosis?

 2. Use the History and Physical and pages 839-840 in your textbook to complete the table below.

Sign/Symptom	Mild Preeclampsia	Severe Preeclampsia	Kelly Brady on Admission
Blood pressure			
Proteinuria			
Headache			
Reflexes			
Visual problems			
Epigastric pain			

• Click on **Physician's Orders** and find the admitting physician's orders on Tuesday at 1030.

3. What tests/procedures did Kelly Brady's physician order to confirm the diagnosis of severe preeclampsia?

• Click on **Physician's Notes**.
• Scroll to the note for Wednesday 0730.

4. What subjective and objective data are recorded here that would support the diagnosis of severe preeclampsia?

Kelly Brady's 24-hour urine collection was completed and sent to the lab at 1230.

 • Click on **Laboratory Reports**.

• Scroll to find the Wednesday 1230 results.

5. Below, record the results of Kelly Brady's 24-hour urine collection.

6. Now list all the data you have collected during this exercise that confirm Kelly Brady's diagnosis of severe preeclampsia.

Exercise 2

 CD-ROM Activity

 20 minutes

• Sign in to work at Pacific View Regional Hospital on the Obstetrics Floor for Period of Care 1. (*Note*: If you are already in the virtual hospital from a previous exercise, click on **Leave the Floor** and then **Restart the Program** to get to the sign-in window.)

• From the Patient List, select Kelly Brady, Room 203.

• Click on **Go to Nurses' Station**.

• Click on **203** at the bottom of the screen to go to the patient's room and perform a physical assessment.

• Click on **Take Vital Signs**.

1. Record Kelly Brady's vital signs for 0730 below.

 • Now click on **Patient Care**. To perform a focused assessment, select the various body areas (yellow buttons) and system subcategories (green buttons) as listed in question 2.

2. Record your findings from the focused assessment of Kelly Brady in the table below.

Assessment Area	Kelly Brady's Findings
Head & Neck Sensory	
Neurologic	
Chest Respiratory	
Abdomen Gastrointestinal	
Lower Extremities Neurologic	

Read pages 842-843 in your textbook; then answer questions 3 and 4.

3. The basic pathophysiology present in a woman with preeclampsia is _____ as

   a result of _____. As a result, blood flow to all organs may
   be diminished.

4. Match each of the signs or symptoms below with the preeclampsia-associated pathology it
   indicates. (*Note:* Some letters will be used more than once.)

   _____ Blurred vision/blind spots   a. Generalized vasoconstriction

   _____ Headache   b. Glomerular damage

   _____ Epigastric or right upper quadrant c. Retinal arteriolar spasms
          abdominal pain
                                              d. Hepatic edema/subcapsular hemorrhage
   _____ 4+ reflexes/clonus
                                              e. Increased CNS irritability
   _____ Elevated blood pressure

   _____ Proteinuria/oliguria

Exercise 3

 CD-ROM Activity

 30 minutes

- Sign in to work at Pacific View Regional Hospital on the Obstetrics Floor for Period of Care 3. (*Note*: If you are already in the virtual hospital from a previous exercise, click on **Leave the Floor** and then **Restart the Program** to get to the sign-in window.)
- From the Patient List, select Kelly Brady.
- Click on **Go to Nurses' Station**.

 Read about HELLP syndrome on pages 843-844 in your textbook.

1. Why do you think Kelly Brady had blood drawn at 1230 for an AST measurement and a platelet count?

- Click on **Chart** and then on the chart for Room **203**.
- Click on **Laboratory Reports**.
- Scroll to the report for Wednesday 1230 to locate the results of these tests.

 2. Complete the table below based on your review of the Laboratory Reports and Table 30-3 on page 844 in your textbook.

Test	Wed 1230 Result	Normal for Pregnancy	Value in HELLP
Platelet count			
AST			

- Click on **Return to Nurses' Station**.
- Click on **Patient List**.
- In the far-right column click on **Get Report** for Kelly Brady.

3. Why has Kelly Brady been transferred to labor and delivery?

4. HELLP syndrome is not a separate illness, but a _____.

However, many women with HELLP syndrome are _____ or have only slightly

elevated blood pressure. HELLP syndrome consists of intravascular _____,

_____ enzymes, and _____ count. HELLP syndrome is a

_____, not a _____, diagnosis.

5. What type woman is most likely to develop HELLP syndrome? Which of these characteristics is true of Kelly Brady?

➡ • Click on **Return to Patient List** and then on **Return to Nurses' Station.**
   • Click on **Chart** and then on **203**.
   • Click on **Physician's Notes**.
   • Scroll to the note for Wednesday 1530.

6. What is the physician's plan of care for Kelly Brady, in light of the HELLP syndrome diagnosis?

Assume that you will be the nurse caring for Kelly Brady after her surgery while she is receiving magnesium sulfate. Read about this medication on pages 851-854 in your textbook and then answer question 7.

7. All of the assessments/interventions listed below are part of routine nursing care for a patient with severe preeclampsia. Place an X beside the activities that are performed specifically to assess for magnesium toxicity.

_____ Measure/record urine output.

_____ Measure proteinuria using urine dipstick.

_____ Monitor liver enzyme levels and platelet count.

_____ Monitor for headache, visual disturbances, and epigastric pain.

_____ Assess for decreased level of consciousness.

_____ Assess DTRs.

_____ Weigh daily to assess for edema.

_____ Monitor vital signs, especially respiratory rate.

_____ Dim room lights and maintain a quiet environment.

11

Antepartal Hemorrhagic Disorders

Reading Assignment: Antepartal Hemorrhagic Disorders (Chapter 32)

Patient: Gabriela Valenzuela, Room 205

Goal: Demonstrate an understanding of the identification and management of selected hemorrhagic complications of pregnancy.

Objectives:

- Identify appropriate interventions for managing abruptio placenta.
- Differentiate between the symptoms related to an abruptio placenta and those related to a placenta previa.
- Plan and evaluate essential patient education during the acute phase of diagnosis.

Exercise 1

 CD-ROM Activity

 45 minutes

- Sign in to work at Pacific View Regional Hospital on the Obstetrics Floor for Period of Care 1. (*Note*: If you are already in the virtual hospital from a previous exercise, click on **Leave the Floor** and then **Restart the Program** to get to the sign-in window.)
- From the Patient List, select Gabriela Valenzuela.
- Click on **Go to Nurses' Station**.
- Click on **Chart** and then on **205**.
- Click on **Emergency Department**.

1. What transpired that brought Gabriela Valenzuela to the ED? How long had she waited to actually come to the ED? What was the deciding factor in her coming to the ED?

Read about the incidence and etiology of abruptio placenta in your textbook on page 875.

2. Other than a motor vehicle accident, what could result in or increase the risk for having an abruptio placenta?

3. Differential diagnosis is very important when you are confronted with clinical manifestations that could be evidence of more than one process. Based on Table 31-3 on page 873 of your textbook, compare and contrast abruptio placenta and placenta previa.

Characteristic/Complication	Abruptio Placenta	Placenta Previa
Bleeding		
Shock complication		
Coagulopathy (DIC)		
Uterine tonicity		
Tenderness/pain		
Placenta findings		
Fetal effects		

 4. Based on your review of the ED Record, what grade of abruption does Gabriela Valenzuela have? Provide supporting documentation from your textbook reading. (*Hint*: Review pages 875-876.)

- Click on **Return to Nurses' Station**.
- Click on **205** to go to the patient's room.
- Click on the **Patient Care**.
- Click on **Nurse-Client Interactions**.
- Select and view the video titled **0740: Patient Teaching—Fetal Monitoring**. (*Note*: If this video is not available, check the virtual clock to see whether enough time has elapsed. The video cannot be viewed before its specified time.)

5. Once Gabriela Valenzuela is admitted to the floor, what are her and her husband's concerns? What does the nurse include in her teaching to alleviate those concerns?

Gabriela Valenzuela is at increased risk for early delivery as a result of the abdominal trauma she suffered and the subsequent occurrence of a grade 1 abruptio placenta. She is currently manifesting signs and symptoms of early labor. According to the Physician's Orders she was given a dose of betamethasone and this was to be repeated in 12 hours.

 6. What is the purpose of the administration of betamethasone in this patient's scenario? (*Hint*: Review information on page 877 of the textbook.)

 • Click on **MAR** and review the betamethasone dosage to be given to Gabriela Valenzuela.
• Click on **Return to Room 205**.
• Click on **Medication Room**.
• Click on **Unit Dosage**.
• Click on drawer **205**.
• Click on **Betamethasone** in the upper left corner of the screen.
• Click on **Put Medication on Tray**.
• Click on **Close Drawer**.
• Click on **View Medication Room**.
• Click on **Preparation**.
• Click on **Prepare** and follow the Preparation Wizard's prompts to complete preparation of Gabriela Valenzuela's betamethasone.
• When the Wizard stops asking questions, click **Finish**.
• Click on **Return to Medication Room**.
• Click on **205** to return to the patient's room.
• Click on **Patient Care**.
• Click on **Medication Administration**.
• Click on **Review Your Medications**.
• Click on the tab marked **Prepared**.

7. According to the text box on the right side of your screen, what is the medication name and dosage that you have prepared for Gabriela Valenzuela?

8. How many mg are you giving to Gabriela Valenzuela based on the answer to the previous question? Is this the correct dosage based on the MAR?

 • Click on **Return to Room 205**
• Click on the **Drug** icon in the left-hand corner of the screen.
• To read about betamethasone, either type the drug name in the Search box or scroll through the alphabetic list of medications at the top of the screen.

9. Based on the information provided in the Drug Guide, what is the indication and dosage for pregnant adults?

10. Based on your review of the baseline assessment data in the Drug Guide, what areas need to be assessed in Gabriela Valenzuela's history?

11. Now review the information regarding the administration of this medication. What are three things that need to be taken into consideration when giving this medication in the injection form?

12. What are the five rights of medication administration as they relate to the patient?

You are now ready to complete the medication administration.

- Click on **Return to Room 205**.

- Click on **Check Armband**.

- Within the purple box under the patient's photo, find **Betamethasone**. Click the down arrow next to **Select** and choose **Administer**.

- Follow the Medication Wizard's prompts to administer Gabriela Valenzuela's betamethasone. Click **Yes** when asked whether to document the injection in the MAR.

- When the Wizard stops asking questions, click **Finish**.

- Now click on **Nurse-Client Interactions**.

- Select and view the video titled **0805: Patient Teaching—Abruption**. (*Note*: If this video is not available, check the virtual clock to see whether enough time has elapsed. The video cannot be viewed before its specified time.)

13. According to the video, what will help increase the oxygen supply to the baby and prevent further separation of the placenta?

- Click on **Leave the Floor**.
- Click on **Look at Your Preceptor's Evaluation**.
- Click on **Medication Scorecard** and review the evaluation. How did you do? (*Hint:* For a quick refresher on reading your Medication Scorecard, see page 22 in the **Getting Started** section of this workbook. For a more detailed tour on preparing and administering medications and interpreting your Scorecard, see pages 26-30 and 36-40.)

Exercise 2

 CD-ROM Activity

 30 minutes

- Sign in to work at Pacific View Regional Hospital on the Obstetrics Floor for Period of Care 2. (*Note:* If you are already in the virtual hospital from a previous exercise, click on **Leave the Floor** and then **Restart the Program** to get to the sign-in window.)
- From the Patient List, select Gabriela Valenzuela.
- Click on **Go to Nurses' Station**.
- Click on **Chart**.
- Click on the chart for Room **205**.
- Click on **Diagnostic Reports**.

Gabriela Valenzuela had an ultrasound done on Tuesday to determine the source of the bleeding.

1. What were the findings on the ultrasound?

- Click on the **Laboratory Reports**.

2. What were Gabriela Valenzuela's hemoglobin and hematocrit levels on Tuesday? How do these findings compare with Wednesday's report? Has there been a significant change?

3. According to the textbook information, the hematocrit level needs to be maintained at

_____. *(Hint:* See page 877 in the textbook.)

 Review collaborative care on pages 876 and 877 in the textbook.

4. What clinical manifestations would indicate a worsening in the condition of either the patient or the fetus?

 • Click on **Return to Nurses' Station**.
- Click on **EPR**.
- Click on **Login**.
- Select **205** as the patient's room and **Vital Signs** as the category.
- Using the blue right and left arrows, scroll to review the vital sign findings over the last 12 hours.

5. From 0000 Wednesday until 1200 Wednesday, would you consider Gabriela Valenzuela's condition stable or unstable? State the rationale for your answer.

 • Click on **Exit EPR**
- Click on **205** at the bottom of the screen.
- Click on **Patient Care**.
- Click on **Nurse-Client Interactions**.
- Select and view the video titled **1140: Intervention—Bleeding, Comfort**. Take notes as you watch and listen. (*Note:* If this video is not available, check the virtual clock to see whether enough time has elapsed. The video cannot be viewed before its specified time.)

6. What happened that elicited this interaction? (*Hint:* Review the Nurse's Notes for Wednesday 1140.)

7. What actions did the nurse take during the interaction?

Exercise 3

 CD-ROM Activity

 15 minutes

- Sign in to work at Pacific View Regional Hospital on the Obstetrics Floor for Period of Care 3. (*Note*: If you are already in the virtual hospital from a previous exercise, click on **Leave the Floor** and then **Restart the Program** to get to the sign-in window.)
- From the Patient List, select Gabriela Valenzuela.
- Click on **Go to Nurses' Station**.
- Click on **Kardex** and then on tab **205**.

1. What problem areas have been identified by the nurse related to Gabriela Valenzuela's diagnosis?

2. What is the focus of the outcomes related to the above mentioned problems?

3. Using correct NANDA nursing diagnosis terminology, list four possible nursing diagnoses appropriate for Gabriela Valenzuela at this time.

• Click on **Return to Nurses' Station**.
  • Click on **Chart**.
  • Click on the chart for Room **205**.
  • Click on **Patient Education**.

4. According to the Patient Education sheet in Gabriela Valenzuela's chart, what are the educational goals related to the patient's diagnosis?

• Click on **Nurse's Notes**.

5. What education has been completed by the nurses through Period of Care 3? Include the times and topics discussed.

6. What are some barriers to learning that the nurse may confront with this patient?

7. How can the nurse overcome each of these?

Endocrine and Metabolic Disorders

/OℤƆ **Reading Assignment:** Endocrine and Metabolic Disorders (Chapter 32)

Patient: Stacey Crider, Room 202

Goal: Demonstrate an understanding of the identification and management of selected endocrine complications of pregnancy.

Objectives:

- Identify appropriate interventions for controlling hyperglycemia in a patient with gestational diabetes mellitus (GDM).
- Correctly administer insulin to a patient with GDM.
- Plan and evaluate essential patient teaching for a patient with GDM.

In this lesson you will describe, plan, and evaluate the care of a patient with gestational diabetes.

Exercise 1

  CD-ROM Activity

30 minutes

- Sign in to work at Pacific View Regional Hospital on the Obstetrics Floor for Period of Care 2. (*Note*: If you are already in the virtual hospital from a previous exercise, click on **Leave the Floor** and then **Restart the Program** to get to the sign-in window.)
- From the Patient List, select Stacey Crider.
- Click on **Go to Nurses' Station**.
- Click on **Chart** and then on the chart for Room **202**.
- Click on **History and Physical**.

1. When was Stacey Crider's GDM diagnosed? How has it been managed thus far?

2. Read about risk factors for GDM on page 895 in your textbook and list them below.

→ • Search for evidence of the risk factors for GDM in Stacey Crider in the **History and Physical** and **Admissions** sections of her chart.

3. Which risk factors for GDM are present in Stacey Crider?

4. What does Stacey Crider's physician suspect is the cause of her poorly controlled blood glucose levels? (*Hint*: See Impression, at the end of the History and Physical.)

→ • Click on **Physician's Orders**.

5. Look at Stacey Crider's admission orders. Write down the orders that are related to GDM.

6. Why did Stacey Crider's physician order a hemoglobin A1C test as part of her admission labs? (*Hint*: See page 887 in your textbook.)

On admission, Stacey Crider is in preterm labor. This was treated with magnesium sulfate tocolysis. She was also given a course of betamethasone.

 • Click on **Return to Nurses' Station**.
 • Click on the **Drug** icon in the lower left corner of the screen.
 • Scroll down the drug list and click on **betamethasone**.

   7. How might betamethasone affect Stacey Crider's GDM?

• Click on **Return to Nurses' Station**.
 • Click on **Chart** and then on **202**.
 • Click on **Physician's Notes**.
 • Scroll to the note for Tuesday at 0700.

   8. How does Stacey Crider's physician plan to deal with these potential medication effects?

Stacey Crider's other admission diagnosis is bacterial vaginosis.

• Click on **Return to Nurses' Station**.
 • Click on **202** at the bottom of your screen.
 • Click on **Patient Care** and then on **Nurse-Client Interactions**.
 • Select and view the video titled **1115: Teaching—Diet, Infection**. (*Note*: If this video is not available, check the virtual clock to see whether enough time has elapsed. The video cannot be viewed before its specified time.)

   9. What is the relationship between Stacey Crider's bacterial vaginosis infection and her GDM?

Exercise 2

 CD-ROM Activity

 20 minutes

- Sign in to work at Pacific View Regional Hospital on the Obstetrics Floor for Period of Care 1. (*Note*: If you are already in the virtual hospital from a previous exercise, click on **Leave the Floor** and then **Restart the Program** to get to the sign-in window.)
- From the Patient List, select Stacey Crider.
- Click on **Go to Nurses' Station**.

 Stacey Crider needs her insulin so that she can eat breakfast. Recall that she receives lispro insulin prior to each meal and NPH insulin at bedtime. Read about the differences in these two types of insulin on page 891 in your textbook.

1. Based on your textbook reading, complete the table below. (*Note*: NPH is considered an intermediate-acting insulin.)

Type of Insulin	Onset of Action	Peak	Duration
Lispro			
Intermediate-acting			

- Click on **EPR** and then on **Login**.
- Click on **202** in Patient drop-down menu. Select **Vital Signs** as the category.
- Look at the vital sign assessment documented on Wednesday at 0700.

2. What is Stacey Crider's blood glucose?

- Click on **Exit EPR**.
- Click on **MAR**.
- Click on tab **202**.

3. What is Stacey Crider's prescribed insulin dosage?

- Click on **Return to Nurses' Station**.
- Click on **Chart**.
- Click on **202**.
- Click on **Physician's Orders**.
- Scroll to the orders for Tuesday at 1900.

4. How much insulin should Stacey Crider receive? Why?

 • Click on **Return to Nurses' Station**.
- Click on **Medication Room**.
- Click on **Unit Dosage**.
- Click on drawer **202**.
- Click on **Insulin Lispro**.
- Click on **Put Medication on Tray**.
- Click on **Close Drawer**.
- Click on **View Medication Room**.
- Click on **Preparation**.
- Click on **Prepare** and follow the prompts to complete preparation of Stacey Crider's lispro insulin dose.
- Click on **Return to Medication Room**.

You are almost ready to give Stacey Crider's insulin injection. However, before you do . . .

5. Considering lispro insulin's rapid onset of action, what else should you check before giving Stacey Crider her injection?

Now you're ready!

• Click on Room **202**.
- Click on **Check Armband**.
- Click on **Patient Care**.
- Click on **Medication Administration**.
- **Insulin Lispro** should be listed on the left side of your screen. Click on the down arrow next to **Select** and choose **Administer**.
- Follow the prompts to administer Stacey Crider's insulin injection. Indicate **Yes** to document the injection in the MAR.
- Click on **Leave the Floor**.
- Click on **Look at Your Preceptor's Evaluation**.
- Click on **Medication Scorecard**. How did you do?

Exercise 3

  CD-ROM Activity

20 minutes

- Sign in to work at Pacific View Regional Hospital on the Obstetrics Floor for Period of Care 3. (*Note*: If you are already in the virtual hospital from a previous exercise, click on **Leave the Floor** and then **Restart the Program** to get to the sign-in window.)
- From the Patient List, select Stacey Crider.
- Click on **Go to Nurses' Station**.
- Click on **Chart** and then on the chart for Room **202**.
- Click on **Patient Education**.

Stacey Crider will likely be discharged home soon. Review her Patient Education record to determine her learning needs in relation to GDM.

1. List the educational goals for Stacey Crider regarding GDM.

 Read the section on Antepartum Care on pages 896-898 in your textbook.

2. Which of Stacey Crider's educational goals would apply to all women with GDM?

3. Which of Stacey Crider's educational goals would *not* apply to all women with GDM? Support your answer.

→ • Click on **Nurse's Notes** and scroll to the note for 0600 Wednesday.

4. How did the nurse describe Stacey Crider's ability to give her own insulin injection at that time?

→ • Click again on **Patient Education**.

5. What teaching has already been done with this patient on Wednesday in regard to GDM?

→ • Click on **Nurse's Notes** and scroll to the note for 1200 Wednesday.

6. Do you think today's initial teaching on insulin administration was effective? Support your answer using objective documentation from the nurse's note.

Use the information you have obtained from the Patient Education form and the Nurse's Notes to answer the following questions.

7. Stacey Crider needs to know all of the following information. Which topic(s) would you choose to work on with her during this period of care?

_____ Verbalize appropriate food choices and portions.

_____ Demonstrate good technique when administering insulin

_____ Demonstrate good technique with self-monitoring of blood glucose.

_____ Recognize hyper- and hypoglycemia and how to treat each.

8. Give a rationale for your answer.

9. Which topic do you think Stacey Crider would choose to work on during this period of care?

_____ Verbalize appropriate food choices and portions.

_____ Demonstrate good technique when administering insulin.

_____ Demonstrate good technique with self-monitoring of blood glucose.

_____ Recognize hyper- and hypoglycemia and how to treat each.

10. Give a rationale for your answer.

Read the section on Postpartum Care on page 898 in your textbook. Stacey Crider has a significant risk for developing glucose intolerance later in life.

11. What advice would you give Stacey Crider to reduce this risk?

12. After delivery, what medical follow-up would you advise for Stacey Crider?

13. Could Stacey Crider's GDM affect her baby after birth? Explain.

Medical-Surgical Problems in Pregnancy

 Reading Assignment: Medical-Surgical Problems in Pregnancy (Chapter 33)

Patients: Maggie Gardner, Room 204
Gabriela Valenzuela, Room 205

Goal: Demonstrate an understanding of the identification and management of selected medical-surgical problems in pregnancy.

Objectives:

- Identify appropriate interventions for managing selected medical-surgical problems in pregnancy.
- Plan and evaluate essential patient education during the acute phase of diagnosis.

Exercise 1

 CD-ROM Activity

🕐 10 minutes

- Sign in to work at Pacific View Regional Hospital on the Obstetrics Floor for Period of Care 1. (*Note*: If you are already in the virtual hospital from a previous exercise, click on **Leave the Floor** and then **Restart the Program** to get to the sign-in window.)
- From the Patient List, select Gabriela Valenzuela.
- Click on **Go to Nurses' Station**.
- Click on **Chart** and then on the chart for Room **205**.
- Click on **History and Physical**.

 Review material regarding cardiac problems during pregnancy on pages 905-908 in the textbook.

1. According to the textbook, 1% of pregnancies are complicated with heart disease. In the History and Physical for Gabriela Valenzuela, what does the physician note as her cardiac problem?

2. Mitral valve disease is one of the most common causes of cardiac disease in pregnant women.
   a. True
   b. False

3. According to the History and Physical, what cardiac symptoms does Gabriela Valenzuela exhibit now that she is pregnant?

4. Based on your textbook reading, why do pregnant women with cardiac disorders have problems during their pregnancy?

5. What abnormal assessment finding is noted in the History and Physical that would be associated with Gabriela Valenzuela's cardiac disorder?

Exercise 2

 CD-ROM Activity

 20 minutes

 Autoimmune disorders encompass a wide variety of disorders that can be disruptive to the pregnancy process. Maggie Gardner in Room 204 has been admitted to rule out lupus. The following activities will explore the various aspects of this autoimmune disorder. First, review pages 925-926 in your textbook regarding systemic lupus erythematosus (SLE).

- Sign in to work at Pacific View Regional Hospital on the Obstetrics Floor for Period of Care 1. (*Note*: If you are already in the virtual hospital from a previous exercise, click on **Leave the Floor** and then **Restart the Program** to get to the sign-in window.)
- From the Patient List, select Maggie Gardner.
- Click on **Go to Nurses' Station**.
- Click on **Chart** and then on the chart for Room **204**.
- Click on **History and Physical**.

1. Based on Maggie Gardner's History and Physical, what information would correlate to a diagnosis of SLE?

2. According to the textbook, what is most often the presenting symptom of this disease during pregnancy?

- Click on **Return to Nurses' Station**.
- Click on Room **204** at the bottom of the screen.
- Click on **Patient Care**.
- Click on **Physical Assessment**.
- Click on various body areas (yellow buttons) and system subcategories (green buttons) to perform a head-to-toe assessment of Maggie Gardner. (*Hint:* Take notes during your assessment based on question 3 and 4.)

3. Based on your head-to-toe assessment, list four abnormal findings that are related to Maggie Gardner's diagnosis.

- Click on **Chart** and then on **204**.
- Click on **Patient Education**.

4. Based on your physical assessment, the information from the Patient Education section of the chart, and the fact that this is a new diagnosis for the patient, list three areas of teaching that need to be completed with this patient.

Exercise 3

 CD-ROM Activity

 35 minutes

- Sign in to work at Pacific View Regional Hospital on the Obstetrics Floor for Period of Care 3. (*Note*: If you are already in the virtual hospital from a previous exercise, click on **Leave the Floor** and then **Restart the Program** to get to the sign-in window.)
- From the Patient List, select Maggie Gardner.
- Click on **Go to Nurses' Station**.
- Click on **Chart**.

- Click on the chart for Room **204**.
- Click on the **Consultations** tab.
- Review the Rheumatology Consult.

1. List four things that the rheumatologist notes in her impressions regarding specific findings that are associated with a diagnosis of SLE for Maggie Gardner.

→ - Click on **Diagnostic Reports**.

2. Maggie Gardner had an ultrasound done prior to the consult with the rheumatologist. What were the findings as they relate to SLE? What were the follow-up recommendations? (*Hint*: See Impressions section.)

3. What is the rheumatologist's plan regarding laboratory/diagnostics to gain a definitive diagnosis?

4. According to the Rheumatology Consult, what is the plan regarding medications (immediate need)?

• Click on **Return to Nurses' Station**
- Click on the **Drug** icon in the lower left corner of the screen.
- Find the Drug Guide profile of prednisone. (*Hint:* You can type the drug name in the Search box or scroll through the alphabetic list of drugs at the top of the screen.)

5. What does Maggie Gardner need to be taught regarding this medication?

 • Click on **Return to Nurses' Station**.
- Click on Room **204**.
- Click on **Patient Care**.
- Click on **Nurse-Client Interactions**.
- Select and view the video titled **1530: Disease Management**. (*Note*: If this video is not available, check the virtual clock to see whether enough time has elapsed. The video cannot be viewed before its specified time.)

6. During this video clip, the nurse provides Maggie Gardner with information regarding her disease. What two things does the nurse note that are important aspects of the patient's disease management during pregnancy?

7. What medication, ordered by the rheumatologist, will assist in the blood flow to the placenta? How?

8. What key component does the nurse identify for Maggie Gardner that will assist in maintaining a healthy pregnancy?

9. What excuse does Maggie Gardner give for not keeping previous doctor's appointments? (*Hint:* This information is also found in the Nursing Admission in the chart.)

Exercise 4

 CD-ROM Activity

 15 minutes

- Sign in to work at Pacific View Regional Hospital on the Obstetrics Floor for Period of Care 4. (*Note*: If you are already in the virtual hospital from a previous exercise, click on **Leave the Floor** and then **Restart the Program** to get to the sign-in window.)
- From the Nurses' Station, click on **Chart**.
- Click on **204** to open Maggie Gardner's chart.
- Click on **Laboratory Reports**.

1. The results are now available for the following laboratory tests that were ordered in Period of Care 2. What are the findings?

Laboratory Test	Result
C3	
C4	
CH50	
RPR	
ANA Titer	
Anticardiolipin	
Anti-sm; Anti-DNA; Anti–SSA	
Anti-SSB	
Anti-RVV; Antiphospholipid	

→ • Click on **Consultations** and review the Rheumatology Consult.

2. The lab findings you recorded in question 1 are definitive for the diagnosis of SLE. According to the textbook and the Rheumatology Consult, what is the plan to manage this disease once the baby is delivered?

→ • Click on **Nurse's Notes.**

3. By Period of Care 4, Maggie Gardner has been provided with education regarding various aspects of her disease process, testing, and hospital procedures. Based on your review of the Nurse's Notes for Wednesday, what has she been specifically taught? Include the time each instruction took place.

4. Using correct NANDA nursing diagnosis terminology, write three possible nursing diagnoses for Maggie Gardner.

5. SLE requires long-term management because patients will experience remissions and exacerbations. What step did the rheumatologist take with Maggie Gardner to begin the long-term relationship that will be required to ensure a healthy outcome?

Mental Health Disorders and Substance Abuse

 Reading Assignment: Mental Health Disorders and Substance Abuse (Chapter 35)

Patients: Kelly Brady, Room 203
Maggie Gardner, Room 204
Laura Wilson, Room 206

Goal: Demonstrate an understanding of the identification and management of selected mental health or substance abuse issues in pregnant women.

Objectives:

- Identify signs and symptoms of depression and anxiety in selected patients.
- Discuss the use of pharmacotherapy for treating depression and anxiety in pregnant and lactating patients.
- Assess and plan care for a substance abusing woman with a term pregnancy.

In this lesson you will assess and plan care for three pregnant women, all of whom have mental health or substance abuse problems.

Exercise 1

 CD-ROM Activity

20 minutes

- Sign in to work at Pacific View Regional Hospital on the Obstetrics Floor for Period of Care 1. (*Note*: If you are already in the virtual hospital from a previous exercise, click on **Leave the Floor** and then **Restart the Program** to get to the sign-in window.)
- From the Patient List, select Kelly Brady.
- Click on **Go to Nurses' Station**.

 Read about Mood Disorders on pages 960-962 in your textbook.

1. List signs and symptoms associated with major depression.

2. In order to be diagnosed with _____, at least

   _____ of the signs/symptoms listed in question 1 must be present

   _____.

3. List risk factors for developing depression in pregnancy.

➤ • Click on **Go to Nurses' Station**
  • Click on **Chart** and then on **203**.
  • Click on **Mental Health** and review the Psychiatric/Mental Health Assessment.

4. List Kelly Brady's signs/symptoms of major depression.

5. Does Kelly Brady meet the criteria for a diagnosis of major depression?

• Click on **Consultations**.
- Scroll to review the Psychiatric Consult, completed Tuesday at 1500.

6. Of the risk factors for developing depression during pregnancy listed in question 3, which are present in Kelly Brady's situation?

7. Using information from the Psychiatric Consult, list data that confirm the presence of the risk factors listed in question 6.

8. What is the management plan for Kelly Brady's depression recommended by the psychiatric consultant?

Read the section on Antidepressant Medications on pages 961-962 in your textbook.

9. What is the drug classification for paroxetine (Paxil)?

10. Kelly Brady plans to breastfeed her baby. How would you counsel her in regard to taking paroxetine (Paxil) while nursing? (*Hint*: Read the section on Medications and Breastfeeding on pages 776-777 in your textbook.)

 11. What suggestions would you give Kelly Brady to help prevent the development of postpartum depression? (*Hint*: See the Teaching for Self-Care box on page 975 in the textbook.)

Exercise 2

 CD-ROM Activity

 20 minutes

- Sign in to work at Pacific View Regional Hospital on the Obstetrics Floor for Period of Care 1. (*Note*: If you are already in the virtual hospital from a previous exercise, click on **Leave the Floor** and then **Restart the Program** to get to the sign-in window.)
- From the Patient List, select Maggie Gardner.
- Click on **Go to Nurses' Station**
- Click on **Chart** and then on the chart for Room **204**.
- Click on **Nursing Admission**.

1. What are Maggie Gardner's admission diagnoses?

2. What seems to be the major cause of Maggie Gardner's anxiety?

3. Is Maggie Gardner's anxiety currently affecting her lifestyle? Support your answer using data from the Nursing Admission.

→ • Click on **History and Physical**.
  • Scroll to the OB History on page 2 of the History and Physical.

4. List Maggie Gardner's obstetric history, using the GTPAL format.

5. Based on Maggie Gardner's previous pregnancy history, why do you think she might be especially anxious at this particular time in her pregnancy?

→ • Click on **Physician's Orders**.
  • Scroll to the admission orders for Tuesday at 2115.

6. Identify the medication and dosage ordered specifically to treat Maggie Gardner's anxiety.

7. What important information is missing from the order in question 6? If you were the nurse caring for Maggie Gardner, how could you obtain this information?

• Click on **Return to Nurses' Station**.
- Click on **204** to go to the patient's room.
- Click on **Patient Care** and then on **Nurse-Client Interactions**.
- Select and view the video titled **0745: Evaluation—Efficacy of Drugs**. (*Note*: If this video is not available, check the virtual clock to see whether enough time has elapsed. The video cannot be viewed before its specified time.)

8. How does Maggie Gardner describe her present emotional state?

9. Does Maggie Gardner believe the buspirone is helping to decrease her anxiety? Why or why not?

10. How does the nurse explain buspirone's effectiveness?

 • Click on the **Drug** icon in the lower left corner of the screen.
- Scroll down the drug list and click on **buspirone**.

11. Is Maggie Gardner's buspirone dosage appropriate?

12. Scroll down to read the Patient Teaching section in the Drug Guide. Based on this information, do you agree with the nurse's explanation about buspirone's effectiveness in the 0745 video? If not, how would you counsel Maggie Gardner about the effectiveness of this medication?

Exercise 3

CD-ROM Activity

20 minutes

- Sign in to work at Pacific View Regional Hospital on the Obstetrics Floor for Period of Care 2. (*Note*: If you are already in the virtual hospital from a previous exercise, click on **Leave the Floor** and then **Restart the Program** to get to the sign-in window.)

- From the Patient List, select Laura Wilson.
- Click on **Go to Nurses' Station**.
- Click on **Chart** and then on the chart for Room **206**.
- Click on **Nursing Admission**.

1. Complete the table by documenting Laura Wilson's use of alcohol and recreational drugs, based on your review of the Nursing Admission.

Substance	Reported Use
Tobacco	
Alcohol	
Marijuana	
Crack cocaine	

 Read about tobacco, alcohol, marijuana, and cocaine in the Substance Abuse During Pregnancy section on pages 964-966 in your textbook.

2. For each pregnancy-related risk listed in the table below, place an X under the substance(s) thought to be associated with that risk.

Pregnancy-Related Risk	Tobacco	Alcohol	Marijuana	Cocaine
Ectopic pregnancy				
Miscarriage				
Premature rupture of membranes				
Preterm birth				
Placenta previa				
Abruptio placentae				
Chorioamnionitis				
Fetal alcohol syndrome (FAS)				
Fetal alcohol effects (FAE)				
Hypertension				
Stillbirth				
Anemia				
Fetal abnormalities				

➔ • Click on **Return to Nurses' Station**.
  • Click on **206** at the bottom of the screen.
  • Click on **Patient Care** and then on **Nurse-Client Interactions**.
  • Select and view the video titled **1115: Teaching—Effects of Drug Use**. (*Note*: If this video is not available, check the virtual clock to see whether enough time has elapsed. The video cannot be viewed before its specified time.)

3. Does Laura Wilson consider herself to be addicted? Support your answer with comments from the video.

4. How does Laura Wilson think her drug use will affect her baby?

5. According to the nurse in the video, how might Laura Wilson's drug use affect the baby?

📖 Read the section on Plan of Care and Intervention on pages 969-971 in your textbook.

6. Assume that you are the nurse caring for Laura Wilson today. Which interventions to deal with Laura Wilson's drug use would be most appropriate at this time?

_____ Talk with Laura Wilson in a manner that conveys caring and concern.

_____ Urge Laura Wilson to begin a drug treatment program today.

_____ Explain to Laura Wilson that she may lose custody of her baby if her drug use continues.

_____ Involve other members of the health care team in Laura Wilson's care.

7. Explain your choice(s) in question 6.

Labor and Birth Complications

📖 **Reading Assignment:** Labor and Birth Complications (Chapter 36)

Patients: Dorothy Grant, Room 201
Stacey Crider, Room 202
Kelly Brady, Room 203
Gabriela Valenzuela, Room 205

Goal: Demonstrate an understanding of the identification and management of selected labor and birth complications.

Objectives:

- Assess and identify signs and symptoms present in the patient with preterm labor.
- Describe appropriate nursing care for the patient in preterm labor.
- Develop a birth plan to meet the needs of the preterm infant.

In this lesson you will compare and contrast the care of four patients, all of whom are treated for preterm labor and/or will deliver preterm infants.

Exercise 1

 CD-ROM Activity

 20 minutes

- Sign in to work at Pacific View Regional Hospital on the Obstetrics Floor for Period of Care 2. (*Note*: If you are already in the virtual hospital from a previous exercise, click on **Leave the Floor** and then **Restart the Program** to get to the sign-in window.)
- From the Patient List, select Dorothy Grant and Gabriela Valenzuela.
- Click on **Go to Nurses' Station**.
- Click on **Chart** and then on **201** for Dorothy Grant's chart.
- Click on **History and Physical**.

1. Using the information found in the History and Physical section, complete the table below for Dorothy Grant.

Patient	Weeks Gestation	Reason for Admission
Dorothy Grant		

- Click on **Return to Nurses' Station**.
- Now click again on **Chart**; this time, select **205** for Gabriela Valenzuela's chart.
- Click on **History and Physical**.

2. Using the information found in the History and Physical section, complete the table below for Gabriela Valenzuela.

Patient	Weeks Gestation	Reason for Admission
Gabriela Valenzuela		

- Click on **Return to Nurses' Station**.
- Click on **201** at the bottom of the screen to go to Dorothy Grant's room.
- Click on **Patient Care**.
- Click on **Physical Assessment**.
- Click on **Pelvic** and then on **Reproductive**.

3. Complete the table below with the results of Dorothy Grant's initial cervical examination.

Patient	Time	Dilation	Effacement	Station
Dorothy Grant				

- Click on **Return to Nurses' Station**.
- Click on **205** to go to Gabriela Valenzuela's room.
- Click on **Patient Care**.
- Click on **Physical Assessment**.
- Click on **Pelvic** and then on **Reproductive**.

4. Record the results of Gabriela Valenzuela's initial cervical examination in the table below.

Patient	Time	Dilation	Effacement	Station
Gabriela Valenzuela				

Read the section on Early Recognition and Diagnosis of preterm labor on pages 987-988 in your textbook.

5. What criteria are necessary in order to make a diagnosis of preterm labor?

6. As of Wednesday at 0800, would you consider both these patients to be in preterm labor? Give a rationale for your answer.

 Read the section on Tocolysis on pages 990-994 in your textbook to answer the following questions.

7. Would you recommend tocolytic therapy for Gabriela Valenzuela? Support your answer.

8. Match each of the medications below with the description of how it works as a tocolytic agent. (Letters may be used more than once.)

_____ Magnesium sulfate

_____ Nifedipine (Procardia)

_____ Ritodrine (Yutopar)

_____ Terbutaline (Brethine)

_____ Indomethacin (Indocin)

a. Inhibits calcium from entering smooth muscle cells, thus relaxing uterine contractions.

b. Relaxes uterine smooth muscle as a result of stimulation of beta$_2$ receptors on uterine smooth muscle.

c. Exact mechanism unclear, but promotes relaxation of smooth muscles

d. Suppresses preterm labor by blocking the production of prostaglandins.

Exercise 2

 CD-ROM Activity

 30 minutes

- Sign in to work at Pacific View Regional Hospital on the Obstetrics Floor for Period of Care 1. (*Note*: If you are already in the virtual hospital from a previous exercise, click on **Leave the Floor** and then **Restart the Program** to get to the sign-in window.)
- From the Patient List, select Stacey Crider.
- Click on **Get Report**.

Stacey Crider was admitted yesterday in preterm labor and placed on magnesium sulfate. Her other admission diagnoses were bacterial vaginosis and gestational diabetes with poorly controlled blood glucose levels.

1. What is Stacey Crider's current status in regard to preterm labor?

→ • Click on **Return to Patient List**; then click **Go to Nurses' Station**.
  • Click on **Chart** and then on the chart for Room **202**.
  • Click on **Physician's Orders**.
  • Scroll to the orders for Wednesday at 0715.

2. Which of these orders relate specifically to Stacey Crider's diagnosis of preterm labor?

→ • Scroll to the orders for Wednesday at 0730.

3. What medication changes are ordered?

Read about terbutaline and nifedipine in Table 36-1 (pages 992-993) in your textbook.

4. Why do you think Stacey Crider's physician changed his orders so quickly?

→ • Click on **Return to Nurses' Station**.
  • Click on **202** at the bottom of the screen.
  • Inside the patient's room, click on **Take Vital Signs**.

5. What are Stacey Crider's current vital signs?

Temperature

Pulse

Respirations

Blood pressure

6. Which of these parameters provides the most important information you would need prior to giving Stacey Crider's nifedipine dose? Why? (*Hint*: Read about nifedipine on pages 991 and 994 in your textbook.)

Like Dorothy Grant and Kelly Brady, Stacey Crider is also receiving betamethasone.

 Read about Promotion of Fetal Lung Maturity in your textbook on pages 994-995. Answer the following questions.

7. Why are all three of these patients receiving antenatal glucocorticoid therapy?

8. What other benefit does this class of medication seem to provide for preterm infants?

 • Click on **MAR**.
  • Click on tab **202**.

9. What is Stacey Crider's prescribed betamethasone dosage?

 10. How does this dosage compare with the recommended dosage listed in the Antenatal Gluco-corticoid Therapy Medication Guide on page 995 of your textbook?

 • Click on **Return to Nurses' Station**.
  • Click on **Medication Room**.
  • Click on **Unit Dosage**.
  • Click on drawer **202**.
  • Click on **Betamethasone**.
  • Click on **Put Medication on Tray**.
  • Click on **Close Drawer**.
  • Click on **View Medication Room**.

- Click on **Preparation**.
- Click on **Prepare** and follow the preparation Wizard's prompts to complete preparation of Stacey Crider's betamethasone dose.
- Click on **Return to Medication Room**.
- Click on **202** to return to Stacey Crider's room.
- Click on **Check Armband**.
- Click on **Check Allergies**.
- Click on **Patient Care**.
- Click on **Medication Administration**.
- Find **Betamethasone** listed on the left side of your screen. To its right, click on the down arrow next to **Select** and choose **Administer**.
- Follow the Administration Wizard's prompts to administer Stacey Crider's betamethasone injection. Indicate **Yes** to document the injection in the MAR.
- Click on **Leave the Floor**.
- Click on **Look at Your Preceptor's Evaluation**.
- Click on **Medication Scorecard**. How did you do?

Exercise 3

 CD-ROM Activity

 30 minutes

- Sign in to work at Pacific View Regional Hospital on the Obstetrics Floor for Period of Care 4. (*Note*: If you are already in the virtual hospital from a previous exercise, click on **Leave the Floor** and then **Restart the Program** to get to the sign-in window.)
- Click on **Chart**.
- Click on **201** for Dorothy Grant's chart.
- Click on **Nurse's Notes**.
- Scroll to the note for Wednesday 1815.

1. Despite receiving terbutaline for tocolysis, Dorothy Grant's labor continues to progress. What are the findings from her cervical examination at this time?

 • Scroll to the note for Wednesday 1840. It states that Dorothy Grant is being prepped for delivery.

2. If you were the nurse caring for Dorothy Grant during delivery, what special preparations would you make to care for the baby immediately after birth?

→ • Click on **Return to Nurses' Station**.
  • Click again on **Chart**, but this time choose **205** for Gabriela Valenzuela's chart.
  • Click on **Physician's Notes**.
  • Scroll to the note for Wednesday 0800.

  3. What is the anticipated outcome of Gabriela Valenzuela's labor, according to this note?

→ • Scroll to the notes for Wednesday 1415 and 1455.

  4. What preparations have been made during the day for the birth of Gabriela Valenzuela's baby?

📖 Read the information on cesarean birth found on pages 1014-1021 in your textbook.

→ • Click on **Return to Nurses' Station**.
  • Once again, click on **Chart**; select **203** for Kelly Brady's chart.
  • Click on **Physician's Notes**.
  • Scroll to the note for Wednesday 1530.

Kelly Brady was admitted yesterday with severe preeclampsia at 26 weeks gestation. Her preeclampsia is now worsening.

  5. Why does her physician now recommend immediate delivery?

  6. What general risks related to cesarean section does Kelly Brady's physician discuss with her?

  7. Because of Kelly Brady's early gestational age (26 weeks), her physician anticipates a classical uterine incision. How will this type of incision affect Kelly Brady's birth options in future pregnancies?

• Click on **Physician's Orders**.
  • Scroll to the orders for Wednesday 1540.

8. List the orders to be carried out prior to Kelly Brady's surgery. State the purpose of each.

Order	Purpose

9. Can you think of other common preoperative procedures? List them below. (*Hint*: Refer to a basic Medical-Surgical textbook for ideas if you need help!)

Newborn Complications

/OᴿⱭ **Reading Assignment:** Acquired Problems of the Newborn (Chapter 38)
Nursing Care of the High-Risk Newborn (Chapter 40)

Patients: Stacey Crider, Room 202
Kelly Brady, Room 203
Gabriela Valenzuela, Room 205
Laura Wilson, Room 206

Goal: Demonstrate an understanding of the identification and management of selected common complications of newborns.

Objectives:

- Describe commonly occurring problems of infants of diabetic mothers.
- List nursing interventions related to hypoglycemia in infants of diabetic mothers.
- Identify risk factors for development of early-onset Group B strep infection and HIV infection.
- Describe common signs and symptoms of early-onset Group B strep infection.
- List nursing interventions for preventing transmission of the HIV virus to the neonate.
- Identify signs and symptoms of in-utero drug exposure in the neonate.
- Identify common problems found in extremely low-birth-weight infants.

In this lesson you will plan care for four newborns, all of whom are considered high-risk for some reason.

Exercise 1

 CD-ROM Activity

 20 minutes

- Sign in to work at Pacific View Regional Hospital on the Obstetrics Floor for Period of Care 4. (*Note*: If you are already in the virtual hospital from a previous exercise, click on **Leave the Floor** and then **Restart the Program** to get to the sign-in window.)
- Click on **Chart** and then on **202** for Stacey Crider's chart.
- Click on **History and Physical**.
- Scroll to History of Present Illness.

1. When was Stacey Crider's gestational diabetes diagnosed?

2. How was Stacey Crider's gestational diabetes managed?

➤ • Click on **Nursing Admission** and scroll to Diagnosis on page 1.

3. What was the status of Stacey Crider's gestational diabetes when she was admitted to the hospital at 27 weeks gestation?

Assume that Stacey Crider has given birth and you are now the nurse caring for Baby Crider. Read the section on Infants of Diabetic Mothers on pages 1056-1059 in your textbook.

4. Listed below are problems often seen in infants of diabetic mothers. Match each problem with the mechanism(s) responsible for that complication. (Answers may be used more than once.)

_____ Congenital anomalies		a. Episodes of ketoacidosis
_____ Macrosomia		b. Fetal hyperinsulinemia
_____ Hypoglycemia		c. Maternal hyperglycemia
_____ Small-for-gestational-age (SGA) infant		d. Fluctuations in maternal blood glucose levels
_____ Respiratory distress syndrome		e. Maternal severe vascular disease

LESSON 16—NEWBORN COMPLICATIONS **155**

5. _____ is defined as a blood glucose level less than 40 mg/dl in a term infant.

   Hypoglycemia most frequently manifests _____. Signs of

   hypoglycemia include _____, _____, _____,

   _____, and, in severe cases, _____.

 Consult the Plan of Care on page 1059 of your textbook.

6. List four nursing interventions to prevent or manage hypoglycemia in Baby Crider.

Exercise 2

 CD-ROM Activity

 30 minutes

Gabriela Valenzuela was admitted at 34 weeks gestation with vaginal bleeding and uterine contractions following a MVA. Her labor progressed throughout the day on Wednesday, and vaginal delivery is expected.

• Sign in to work at Pacific View Regional Hospital on the Obstetrics Floor for Period of Care 4. (*Note*: If you are already in the virtual hospital from a previous exercise, click on **Leave the Floor** and then **Restart the Program** to get to the sign-in window.)
• Click on **MAR**, and then on tab **205** for Gabriela Valenzuela's records.

1. What medication has Gabriela Valenzuela been receiving today for Group B streptococcus prophylaxis?

→ • Click on **Return to Nurses' Station**.
• Click on **Chart** and then on the chart for Room **205**.
• Click on **Nurse's Notes**.
• Scroll to the note for Wednesday 1820.

2. What are the findings of Gabriela Valenzuela's cervical exam at this time?

Copyright © 2006 by Mosby, Inc. All rights reserved.

Assume that Gabriela Valenzuela does give birth today. Read the Group B Streptococcus section on page 1056 in your textbook.

3. All of the following are risk factors for the development of early-onset GBS infection. Place an X beside the risk factor that you know would apply to Baby Valenzuela.

_____ Low birth weight

_____ Preterm birth

_____ Rupture of membranes of more than 18 hours

_____ Maternal fever

_____ Previous infant with GBS infection

_____ Maternal GBS bacteriuria

_____ Multiple gestation

4. GBS infection most commonly manifests _____. GBS

infection usually results from _____ transmission from the _____.

5. If you were the nurse caring for Baby Valenzuela, what signs/symptoms might you see if the baby developed early-onset GBS?

Laura Wilson is a G1 P0 at 37 weeks gestation who is also HIV-positive. She was admitted last night with fever, vomiting, and diarrhea to rule out acute abdomen and pyelonephritis. During the day on Wednesday, Laura Wilson began having mild uterine contractions.

→ • From the Nurses' Station, click on **Chart** and then on the chart for Room **206**.
  • Click on **Physician's Notes**.
  • Scroll to the note for Wednesday at 0830.

6. Below, record Laura Wilson's HIV-related lab values.

CD4 count

HIV-1 RNA count

→ • Click on **Physician's Orders**.
  • Scroll to the admission orders for Tuesday at 2130.

7. What is Laura Wilson's current antiretroviral drug regimen?

→ • Click on **Nurse's Notes**.

  • Scroll to the note for Wednesday 1830

8. What event occurred at 1815?

9. Is Laura Wilson in labor at this time? Support your answer.

Laura Wilson is transferred to labor and delivery to give birth. Assume that she does give birth today. Read the section on Human Immunodeficiency Virus and Acquired Immunodeficiency Syndrome on pages 1065-1067 in your textbook.

10. List factors that, if present, would increase the risk for transmission of HIV to Laura Wilson's baby during the birth process. Which risk factor does Laura Wilson have at this time?

11. All infants born to HIV-positive mothers should be assumed to be _____. The

    accuracy of HIV testing in infants varies according to _____ and is

    dependent on _____. The three methods currently used to

    detect HIV in neonates are _____, _____, and

    _____. Testing should be done

    _____, _____, and _____.

12. What is the current testing recommendation of the Centers for Disease Control and Prevention (CDC) in order to make a definitive diagnosis of HIV infection?

13. Assume that you are the nurse caring for Baby Wilson in the newborn nursery. List nursing interventions to decrease the risk for viral transmission to the baby.

_____

Exercise 3

 CD-ROM Activity

 15 minutes

In addition to being HIV-positive, Laura Wilson also has a past and current history of substance abuse.

• Sign in to work at Pacific View Regional Hospital on the Obstetrics Floor for Period of Care 4. (_Note_: If you are already in the virtual hospital from a previous exercise, click on **Leave the Floor** and then **Restart the Program** to get to the sign-in window.)
• Click on **Chart** and then on **206** for Laura Wilson's chart.
• Click on **Nursing Admission**.

1. Complete the chart below with information on Laura Wilson's current use of alcohol and recreational drugs (found on page 4 of the Nursing Admission).

Substance	Reported Use
Alcohol	
Marijuana	
Crack cocaine	

 Read about alcohol, marijuana, and cocaine in the Substance Abuse section on pages 1071-1074 in your textbook.

2. Listed below are problems often seen in infants exposed prenatally to alcohol, marijuana, or cocaine. Indicate the substance(s) thought to be associated with each problem by marking an X in the proper column(s). (*Note:* More than one drug may be associated with each problem.)

Problem	Alcohol	Marijuana	Cocaine
Craniofacial abnormalities			
Decreased birth weight			
Hyperactivity			
Congenital anomalies			
Developmental delay			
Hypersensitivity to noise and external stimuli			
Difficult to console			

3. Fetal alcohol syndrome (FAS) is based on minimal criteria of signs in each of three

   categories: _____,

   _____, and _____. A baby with

   _____ has been affected by prenatal exposure to alcohol but
   does not meet the criteria for FAS.

Read the Nursing Care section on pages 1077-1079 in your textbook.

4. List several appropriate interventions for the nurse assigned to work with Laura Wilson and her newborn.

Exercise 4

 CD-ROM Activity

 20 minutes

Kelly Brady was admitted with severe preeclampsia at 26 weeks gestation. Because of worsening maternal condition, she gives birth on Wednesday by cesarean section.

- Sign in to work at Pacific View Regional Hospital on the Obstetrics Floor for Period of Care 4. (*Note*: If you are already in the virtual hospital from a previous exercise, click on **Leave the Floor** and then **Restart the Program** to get to the sign-in window.)
- Click on **Chart** and then on **203** for Kelly Brady's chart.
- Click on **Diagnostic Reports**.

1. According to the ultrasound done on Tuesday, what is Baby Brady's estimated fetal weight?

 • Click on **Consultations**.
- Review the Neonatology Consult for Wednesday at 0800.

2. List common problems for babies born at 26 weeks gestation at Pacific View Regional Hospital, according to the neonatologist who met with Kelly Brady and her husband.

 Read the section on Preterm Infants: Care Management, Assessment and Nursing Diagnoses on pages 1112-1116 in your textbook.

3. If Baby Brady's actual birth weight is close to her estimated weight, in which weight category will she be placed? Why?

4. Many body systems or functions are likely to be impaired in ELBW infants. Place an X beside the systems or functions that were also addressed by the neonatologist during his consultation with Kelly Brady. (*Hint:* See your answer to question 2.)

_____ Respiratory function

_____ Cardiovascular function

_____ Maintenance of body temperature

_____ CNS function

_____ Maintenance of adequate nutrition

_____ Maintenance of renal function

_____ Maintenance of hematologic status

_____ Resistance to infection

5. List several psychologic tasks that Kelly Brady and/or her husband must accomplish as parents of Baby Brady.

6. Write a nursing diagnosis appropriate for the Bradys, as parents of a premature baby who will have an extended NICU stay. (*Hint*: Consult the Plan of Care on pages 1130-1131 in the textbook.)

7. List several nursing interventions to assist the Bradys in accomplishing the parenting tasks you listed in question 5. (*Hint*: Consult the Plan of Care on pages 1130-1131 in the textbook.)

Grieving the Loss of a Newborn

 Reading Assignment: Grieving the Loss of a Newborn (Chapter 41)

Patient: Maggie Gardner, Room 204

Goal: Demonstrate an understanding of the grieving process and how it relates to coping with a current pregnancy.

Objectives:

- Identify the various types of loss as they relate to a pregnancy.
- Describe the stages and phases of the grieving process.
- Identify various methods of coping exhibited by patients who have experienced the loss of a newborn.

Exercise 1

Writing Activity

 10 minutes

Review pages 1150-1151 in the textbook.

1. Parents may grieve not only the death of a newborn but also the birth of a baby with a

   _____ or _____.

2. List other times that couples may grieve a loss related to pregnancy?

3. Women experience what type of effects if a pregnancy ends early due to miscarriage?

4. Miscarriages occur in _____ of all pregnancies

5. Grief involves _____ and related _____ and _____ responses to a major loss.

6. All women and men who undergo a loss receive the support that they need.
   a. True
   b. False

Exercise 2

CD-ROM Activity

10 minutes

- Sign in to work at Pacific View Regional Hospital on the Obstetrics Floor for Period of Care 4. (*Note*: If you are already in the virtual hospital from a previous exercise, click on **Leave the Floor** and then **Restart the Program** to get to the sign-in window.)
- Click on **Chart** and then on **204** for Maggie Gardner's chart.
- Review the **History and Physical**.

1. How many losses related to pregnancy has Maggie Gardner experienced?

- Click on the **Nursing Admission**.

2. What is the first evidence you find that Maggie Gardner's previous losses are affecting her current pregnancy and care? (*Hint*: Review the first five sections.)

- Click on the **Consultations** tab.

3. To what does Maggie Gardner attribute her inability to have a child?

4. List three therapeutic measures the chaplain can use to assist her through these feelings as part of her grieving process?

5. What did the chaplain accomplish during his time with Maggie Gardner?

Exercise 3

CD-ROM Activity

15 minutes

Review pages 1151-1154 in your textbook.

1. What is grief?

2. What are the four tasks of grief?

3. What are the three phases of grief?

4. Mothers are the focus during the loss of an infant; however, the _____ shares

the _____ level of grief.

5. What response typically emerges during intense grief? Why?

6. List three other emotions that are experienced during the time period of intense grief.

7. During the phase of reorganization, what is the most common question? Explain.

→ • Sign in to work at Pacific View Regional Hospital on the Obstetrics Floor for Period of Care 4. (*Note:* If you are already in the virtual hospital from a previous exercise, click on **Leave the Floor** and then **Restart the Program** to get to the sign-in window.)
   • Click on **Chart** and then on **204**.
   • Review the **History and Physical**.

8. You have now reviewed Maggie Gardner's History and Physical and compared her information with your textbook's discussion of what happens during the reorganization phase. What correlation do you see?

→ • Click on **Consultations**.
   • Scroll down to review the Pastoral Care Spiritual Assessment.

9. Culture and religion play very large roles in how individuals handle a loss. How has Maggie Gardner handled her losses? (*Hint*: See the Spirituality/Faith Factors section of this consult.)

LESSON **18** _____

Medication Administration

_____

Patients: Dorothy Grant, Room 201
Stacey Crider, Room 202
Maggie Gardner, Room 204
Laura Wilson, Room 206

Goal: Correctly administer selected medications to obstetric patients.

Objective:

• Correctly administer selected medications to obstetric patients, observing the Five Rights.

In this lesson you will give medications to selected obstetrics patients, observing the Five Rights.

Exercise 1

 CD-ROM Activity

 30 minutes

Dorothy Grant was admitted at 30 weeks gestation for observation following blunt abdominal trauma (she was kicked in the abdomen). She is bleeding vaginally and may have sustained a placental abruption. Your assignment for this exercise is to give Rho(D) immune globulin to Dorothy Grant.

• Sign in to work at Pacific View Regional Hospital on the Obstetrics Floor for Period of Care 2. (*Note*: If you are already in the virtual hospital from a previous exercise, click on **Leave the Floor** and then **Restart the Program** to get to the sign-in window.)
• From the Patient List, select Dorothy Grant.

Read about Rho(D) immune globulin on page 636 in your textbook.

1. Rho(D) immune globulin is a solution of _____ that contains _____.

   Rho(D) immune globulin is given to _____

   who has had a _____.

   Rho(D) immune globulin prevents sensitization by _____

   _____.

2. All of the following are reasons that Rho(D) immune globulin might be administered. Place an X next to the reason it has been ordered for Dorothy Grant.

   _____ Within 72 hours of giving birth to an Rh-positive infant

   _____ Prophylactically at 28 weeks gestation

   _____ Following an incident or exposure risk that occurs after 28 weeks gestation

   _____ During first trimester pregnancy following miscarriage or elective abortion or ectopic pregnancy

3. List the information about Dorothy Grant that must be determined before giving her Rho(D) immune globulin.

→ • Click on **Go to Nurses' Station**.
   • Click on **Chart** and then on **201**.
   • Click on **Physician's Orders**.
   • Scroll to the orders for Wednesday 0730.

4. Write the physician's order for Rho(D) immune globulin.

5. According to your textbook, is this the correct dosage and route?

→ • Click on **Laboratory Reports**
   • Locate the results for 0245 Wednesday.
   • Scroll down to find the type and screen results.

6. Dorothy Grant's blood type is _____.

7. What additional information do you need? Why? Is that information available?

 • Click on **Return to Nurses' Station**.
- Click on **Medication Room**.
- Click on **Refrigerator**; then click on the refrigerator door to open it.
- Click on **Put Medication on Tray**.
- Click on **Close Door**.
- Click on **View Medication Room**.
- Click on **Preparation**.
- Click on **Prepare** and follow the prompts to complete preparation of this medication.
- Click on **Return to Medication Room**.
- Click on **201** to go to Dorothy Grant's room.
- Click on **Check Armband**.
- Click on **Patient Care**.
- Click on **Medication Administration**.

You are almost ready to give Dorothy Grant's injection. However, before you do . . .

8. Rho(D) immune globulin is often considered a blood product.
   a. True
   b. False

9. Suppose Dorothy Grant tells you that she is a Jehovah's Witness and absolutely refuses to accept blood or blood products. How would you handle the situation?

Now you're ready to administer the medication!

• Click on the down arrow next to **Select**; choose **Administer**.
- Follow the prompts to administer Dorothy Grant's injection. Indicate **Yes** to document the injection in the MAR.
- Click on **Leave the Floor**.
- Click on **Look at Your Preceptor's Evaluation**.
- Click on **Medication Scorecard**. How did you do?

Exercise 2

 CD-ROM Activity

20 minutes

- Sign in to work at Pacific View Regional Hospital on the Obstetrics Floor for Period of Care 1. (*Note*: If you are already in the virtual hospital from a previous exercise, click on **Leave the Floor** and then **Restart the Program** to get to the sign-in window.)
- From the Patient List, select Maggie Gardner.
- Click on **Go to Nurses' Station**.
- Click on the **Chart** and then on **204**.
- Click on the **Nursing Admission**.

1. Maggie Gardner verbalizes anxiety repeatedly throughout the Nursing Admission. What is her primary concern? Why? Provide documentation.

2. Maggie Gardner states that prior to this pregnancy she had a highly adaptive coping mechanism. How does she consider her ability to cope at this point? Why? (*Hint*: See the Coping and Stress Tolerance section in the Nursing Admission.)

 • Click on the **Physician's Orders**

3. What medication has the physician ordered to help Maggie Gardner with her anxiety?

• Click on **Return to Nurses' Station**.
- Click on the **Drug** icon in the lower-left corner of your screen.
- Use the Search box or the scroll bar to find the medication you identified in question 3.
- Review all of the information provided regarding this drug.

4. What is the drug's mechanism of action?

- Click on **Return to Nurses' Station**.
- Click on **204** to go to Maggie Gardner's room.
- Click on **Patient Care**.
- Click on **Nurse-Client Interactions**.
- Select and view the video titled **0745: Evaluation—Efficacy of Drugs**. (*Note*: If this video is not available, check the virtual clock to see whether enough time has elapsed. The video cannot be viewed before its specified time.)

5. According to the nurse, how long will it take for Maggie Gardner to see therapeutic effects? How does this correlate with what you learned in the Teaching Section of the Drug Guide?

Exercise 3

 CD-ROM Activity

 15 minutes

In this exercise, you will administer betamethasone to Stacey Crider, who was admitted to the hospital at 27 weeks gestation in preterm labor.

- Sign in to work at Pacific View Regional Hospital on the Obstetrics Floor for Period of Care 1. (*Note*: If you are already in the virtual hospital from a previous exercise, click on **Leave the Floor** and then **Restart the Program** to get to the sign-in window.)
- From the Patient List, select Stacey Crider.

1. Before preparing Stacey Crider's betamethasone, what do you need to do first?

- Click on **Go to Nurses' Station**.
- Click on **Chart** and then on the chart for Room **202**.
- Click on **Physician's Orders**.
- Scroll until you find the order for betamethasone.

2. After verifying the physician's order, what's your next step?

• Click on **Return to Nurses' Station**.
• Click on **Medication Room**.
• Click on **Unit Dosage**.
• Click on drawer **202**.
• Click on **Betamethasone**.
• Click on **Put Medication on Tray**.
• Click on **Close Drawer**.
• Click on **View Medication Room**.
• Click on **Preparation**.
• Click on **Prepare** and follow the prompts to complete preparation of Stacey Crider's betamethasone dose.
• Click on **Return to Medication Room**.

   3. Now that the medication is prepared, what's your next step?

 • Click on **202** to go to the patient's room.
• Click on **Check Armband**.
• Click on **Check Allergies**.
• Click on **Patient Care**.
• Click on **Medication Administration**.
• Click on the down arrow next to **Select** and choose **Administer**.
• Follow the prompts to administer Stacey Crider's betamethasone injection.

   4. What's the final step in the process?

• If you haven't already, indicate **Yes** to document the injection in the MAR.
• Click on **Leave the Floor**.
• Click on **Look at Your Preceptor's Evaluation**.
• Click on **Medication Scorecard**. How did you do?

Exercise 4

 CD-ROM Activity

30 minutes

- Sign in to work at Pacific View Regional Hospital on the Obstetrics Floor for Period of Care 1. (*Note*: If you are already in the virtual hospital from a previous exercise, click on **Leave the Floor** and then **Restart the Program** to get to the sign-in window.)
- From the Patient List, select Laura Wilson.
- Click on **Go to Nurses' Station**.
- Click on **MAR**.
- Click on the tab for Room **206**.

1. Laura Wilson's medications for Wednesday include several different types of drugs. In the list below, place an X next to the one that is used to treat her HIV-positive status.

    _____ Zidovudine 200 mg po every 8 hours

    _____ Prenatal multivitamin 1 tablet po daily

    _____ Lactated Ringer's 1000 mL IV continuous

- Click on **Return to Nurses' Station**.
- Click on the **Drug** icon in the lower-left conrner of the screen.
- Using the Search box or the scroll bar, find the drug you identified in question 1.

2. What is the drug's mechanism of action?

3. What is the drug's therapeutic effect?

4. Does this medication cross the placenta, or is it distributed in breast milk?

5. What symptoms/side effects of this medication need to be reported to the physician?

6. How should this medication be taken?

7. Your final assignment is to give Laura Wilson the medication that is due at 0800. During these lessons, we have provided you with the detailed instructions on how to give medications. Now it is time for you to fly solo. Don't forget the Five Rights of medication administration . . . and have fun!! Document below how you did.

If you'd like to get more practice, there are other medications that can be given at the beginning of the first three periods of care. Below is a list of the patients, the medications, the routes of administration, and the administration times you can use. As you practice, be sure to select the correct patient when you sign in. That way, you can get a Medication Scorecard for evaluation after you prepare and administer a medication. (*Remember:* If you need help at any time, refer to pages 22, 26-30, and 36-40 in the **Getting Started** section of this workbook.)

Period of Care 1

Room 201, Dorothy Grant

0730/0800

Betamethasone 12 mg IM

Prenatal multivitamin PO

Room 202, Stacey Crider

0800—Prenatal multivitamin PO

Metronidazole 500 mg PO

Betamethasone 12 mg IM

Insulin lispro Sub-Q

Nifedipine 20 mg PO

Room 203, Kelly Brady

0730/0800—Prenatal multivitamin PO

Ferrous sulfate PO

Labetalol hydrochloride 400 mg PO

Nifedipine 10 mg PO

Room 204, Maggie Gardner

0800—Prenatal multivitamin PO

Buspirone hydrochloride 5 mg PO

Room 205, Gabriela Valenzuela

0800—Ampicillin 2 g IV

Betamethasone 12 mg IM

Prenatal multivitamin PO

Room 206, Laura Wilson

0800—Zidovudine 200 g PO

Prenatal multivitamin PO

PERIOD OF CARE 2

Room 201, Dorothy Grant

1200—Rho(D) immune globulin IM

Room 202, Stacey Crider

1200—Insulin lispro Sub-Q

Room 203, Kelly Brady

1130—Betamethasone 12 mg IM

Room 204, Maggie Gardner

1115—Prednisone 40 mg PO

Aspirin 81 mg PO

PERIOD OF CARE 3

Room 204, Maggie Gardner

1500—Buspirone 5 mg PO